This volume provides an introduction to the essential techniques required for studying the molecular biology of brain disease. The approaches and strategies for investigations of gene structure and regulation are described with reference to the molecular genetics of prion and Alzheimer's disease. The effects of aberrant gene regulation can also be examined at the protein level by immunocytochemistry and autoradiography. Improved understanding of basic biology has resulted in new approaches to animal models using transgenic techniques and new therapeutic approaches. The volume is structured to illustrate all these approaches and demonstrate the practice and promise of molecular neuropathology.

Molecular neuropathology

POSTGRADUATE MEDICAL SCIENCE

This important new series is based on the successful and internationally well-regarded specialist training programme at the Royal Postgraduate Medical School in London. Each volume provides an integrated and self-contained account of a key area of medical science, developed in conjunction with the course organisers and including contributions from specially invited authorities.

The aim of the series is to provide biomedical and clinical scientists with a reliable introduction to the theory and to the technical and clinical applications of each topic.

The volumes will be a valuable resource and guide for trainees in the medical and biomedical sciences, and for laboratory-based scientists.

Titles in the series

Radiation protection of patients edited by Richard Wootton

Monoclonal antibodies edited by Mary A. Ritter and Heather M. Ladyman

Image analysis in histology: conventional and confocal microscopy edited by R. Wootton, D. R. Springall and J. M. Polak

Molecular neuropathology

EDITED BY

GARETH W. ROBERTS

*Director, Molecular Neuropathology Department, SmithKline Beecham
Pharmaceuticals, Harlow*

and

JULIA M. POLAK

Professor, Department of Histochemistry, Royal Postgraduate Medical School, London

Published in association with
the Royal Postgraduate Medical School
University of London by

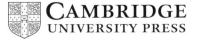 **CAMBRIDGE**
UNIVERSITY PRESS

Published by the Press Syndicate of the University of Cambridge
The Pitt Building, Trumpington Street, Cambridge CB2 1RP
40 West 20th Street, New York, NY 10011-4211, USA
10 Stamford Road, Oakleigh, Melbourne 3166, Australia

© Cambridge University Press 1995

First published 1995

Printed in Great Britain at the University Press, Cambridge

A catalogue record for this book is available from the British Library

Library of Congress cataloguing in publication data

Molecular neuropathology / edited by G. W. Roberts and J. Polak.
    p.   cm. – Postgraduate medical science)
Includes index.
ISBN 0 521 42558 1 (pbk.)
1. Nervous system – Diseases – Molecular aspects.   I. Roberts,
Gareth W.   II. Polak, Julia M.   III. Series.
RC347.M648 1995
616.8′047 – dc20   94-38468 CIP

ISBN 0 521 42558 1   paperback

KT

Contents

Contributors

Harry F. Baker

MRC Comparative Cognition Research Team, Department of Experimental Psychology, Downing Street, Cambridge CB2 3EB, UK

Frances Busfield

Department of Psychiatry, Washington University School of Medicine, 4940 Children's Place, St Louis, MO 63110, USA

John Collinge

Prion Disease Research Group, Department of Biochemistry, St. Mary's Hospital Medical School, Norfolk Place, London W2 1PG, UK

Karen Duff

University of South Florida, Alzheimer Disease Research Labs, MDC14, 3515 E Fletcher Ave, Tampa, FL 33613, USA

Stephen M. Gentleman

Department of Psychiatry and Anatomy, Charing Cross and Westminster Medical School, Dunstan's Road, London W6 8RP, UK

Alison Goate

Department of Psychiatry, Washington University School of Medicine, 4940 Children's Place, St Louis, MO 63110, USA

Paul J. Harrison

Department of Psychiatry, University of Oxford, Warneford Hospital, Oxford OX3 7JX, UK

Corinne Lendon

Department of Psychiatry, Washington University School of Medicine, 4940 Children's Place, St Louis, MO 63110, USA

Jeanette McKenzie

Department of Psychiatry and Anatomy, Charing Cross and Westminster Medical School, Dunstan's Road, London W6 8RP, UK

Mark S. Palmer

Prion Disease Research Group, Department of Biochemistry, St. Mary's Hospital Medical School, Norfolk Place, London W2 1PG, UK

R. Carl A. Pearson   Department of Biomedical Sciences, The
                          University, Sheffield S10 2TN, UK

Rosalind M. Ridley   MRC Comparative Cognition Research Team,
                          Department of Experimental Psychology, Downing
                          Street, Cambridge CB2 3EB, UK

Gareth W. Roberts   Molecular Neuropathology Department,
                          SmithKline Beecham Pharmaceuticals,
                          Coldharbour Road, The Pinnacles, Harlow, Essex
                          CM19 5AD, UK

M. Claire Royston   Department of Psychiatry and Anatomy, Charing
                          Cross and Westminster Medical School, Dunstan's
                          Road, London W6 8RP, UK

Martin D. Stefan   Department of Psychiatry and Anatomy, Charing
                          Cross and Westminster Medical School, Dunstan's
                          Road, London W6 8RP, UK

PART 1

Basic techniques

1

Brain banks

MARTIN D. STEFAN
and M. CLAIRE ROYSTON

Introduction

Definitions

Biological specimen banks in general can be defined as systems 'which will store one or many types of biologic specimens for later analysis from single or multiple studies under conditions which permit efficient retrieval and optimum stability of the samples' (Winn *et al.*, 1990).

Brain banks are a specific type of specimen bank, which as well as collecting, storing and distributing human post-mortem brain tissue, may also be involved in handling brain biopsy material and other tissues such as serum and cerebrospinal fluid (CSF). Many of the considerations that apply to the running of a brain bank are general to all forms of specimen bank, and include legal and ethical issues, diagnosis and classification, technical issues and administration. There are also problems specific to human brain-specimen banks: suitable material is scarce for a number of reasons; technical considerations place significant constraints on the acceptability of potential donor material; the complexities of diagnosis and classification assume great significance; and the long-term nature of brain banking coupled with the rapid rate of advance in neuroscientific research techniques demands that great care be taken in designing technical protocols that allow for the broadest possible repertoire of research methods.

Applications

Brain banks have been important in neuroscience research since the elucidation of the basic pathophysiology of Parkinson's disease. They are of particular importance in the investigation of those severe chronic brain diseases without adequate animal models. The current explosion of interest in Alzheimer's disease and other dementias, and in the so-called 'functional psychoses', schizophrenia and the major mood disorders, is likely to increase demands on the limited resources currently available.

The limitations of a particular brain bank will be determined by the diagnostic and technical protocols deployed. Some irrevocable decisions, for example about preservation techniques and maximum acceptable post-mortem interval, will need to be taken on their inception, and will be dictated by current requirements, but planning for maximum flexibility with regard to unpredictable future research needs is also important and this should not be neglected in the design of protocols.

Ethical and legal considerations

It goes without saying that adherence to the highest ethical standards in research of this nature is paramount. Local ethical committee approval is mandatory, the wording of consent forms must be carefully and sensitively worked out, and clinical confidentiality must be preserved. Brahams (1990) has briefly outlined the legal position pertaining to brain banking in the UK, which is covered by sections of the Human Tissue Act 1961. This makes provision not only for written, or witnessed oral consent on the part of a patient, for the use of organs for research purposes, but also for consent after the patient's death by surviving relatives. The latter is of particular relevance in the collection of control specimens, where prospective consent is unlikely to be feasible. Consent from relatives must also be obtained when a potential donor has agreed to inclusion, if there is any doubt about the informed nature of this consent. Brahams also makes the point that consent forms should be worded in such a way as not to restrict the scope or nature of the research for which the organs may be used. In the US, organ donation comes under the provisions of the Uniform Anatomical Gift Act 1987. Adherence to the highest ethical standards demands the fostering of careful and sensitive contacts with potential donors and their families, and this can only be to the benefit of all concerned.

Diagnosis and classification

Without good clinical or neuropathological diagnostic classification, setting up a brain bank is a waste of time, effort and resources. Diseases can be classified in terms of their aetiology, their pathology, or their clinical features, in general with corresponding diminishing degrees of precision. In the case of brain disease with obvious pathological features (e.g. Alzheimer's), or known aetiology (e.g. CNS manifestations of HIV infection), diagnosis should be a relatively straightforward task; specific laboratory investigations may be available, albeit for a minority of conditions at present, and neuropathological examination should normally form part of the collection or research protocol.

The problem is considerably more complex in the case of the functional psychoses, where diagnosis is at present based entirely on the clinical signs and symptoms elicited from a case. An important decision in the design of a protocol is whether to rely on prospective or retrospective diagnosis. Prospective studies allow for accuracy and detail in the clinical information collected ante-mortem, at the cost of increased timescale and limited sample number. Frequency of follow up will need to be considered, and will be determined by the stability over time of the clinical features of the disease under investigation: thus, research on a rapidly progressive illness such as Alzheimer's disease may require more frequent routine assessment of potential donors than research in schizophrenia, where symptomatology tends towards greater stability, and where changes are more likely to come to clinical attention. In the case of the affective disorders, where brain material from victims of suicide may be used, adequate clinical information may be lacking: Ferrier & Perry (1992) have pointed out the dangers inherent in this approach, particularly with respect to the assumption that the neurobiology of suicide is the same as that of depression. In general, material used should be confined to those individuals who have been in contact with clinical services ante-mortem.

Retrospective studies will allow for a greater sample size, but the quality of clinical information is likely to be compromised to some extent: routine case notes vary in their style and may display a paucity of relevant information. In particular, often only significant positive findings may be recorded, and detailed results of special investigations such as neuropsychological assessments, which may be central to the testing of a specific hypothesis, are less likely to be available.

Diagnostic systems

The standardization of psychiatric diagnosis, and the related issue of the measurement of psychiatric symptoms, holds many pitfalls and requires great care at an early stage in the planning of research involving human brain specimen banks.

Research diagnosis is normally determined by operationalized criteria, which provide an explicit list of features that must be present, together with exclusion criteria. Farmer, McGuffin & Bebbington (1988) have reviewed the advantages as well as the limitations of this approach in the context of schizophrenia. The general effect of operationalizing diagnostic criteria is to improve diagnostic reliability, but no such improvement is necessarily seen for the validity of the diagnosis reached. A trivial illustration of this problem, offered by Farmer *et al.*, would be the inclusion of a diagnostic requirement that for the diagnosis of schizophrenia to be made, subjects must be over 6 foot (180 cm) tall. This could obviously be measured with great reliability, but do nothing for the validity of the diagnosis. More realistically, it is known that different diagnostic criteria may identify populations with quite different clinical and demographic characteristics. Using multiple sets of diagnostic criteria does not necessarily help overcome this problem, and Farmer *et al.* (1992) argue that such systems must not be viewed as a substitute for clinical judgement. Nevertheless, the advantages offered by operationalized criteria such as those contained in

DSM-III-R (American Psychiatric Association, 1987) are of a magnitude that ensures their universal use and widespread acceptance. Less unanimity exists about methods to quantify psychiatric symptoms, which may be extremely subtle and poorly documented in routine casenotes. In these circumstances, the advantages of prospective studies with well-defined protocols for clinical assessment become overwhelming. The use of retrospective clinical data is nevertheless a fact of life for many involved in research using post-mortem brain material, and it would be entirely unrealistic to demand perfection in the quality of clinical data available to them. It would not be unreasonable, however, to expect maximum use to be made of the data that does exist, and medical and treatment histories, details of concurrent illnesses, demographic information, family pedigrees, the results of clinical and laboratory investigations, and full sets of contemporaneous casenotes, should be kept with the pathological material and made available to the researcher.

Technical considerations

There are any number of theoretically good procedures for dissecting and storing a brain, and in view of the unpredictability of future developments in techniques of neurobiological investigation, it would probably be a mistake to aim for standardized protocols (which may have unforeseen limitations) between brain banks (Swaab et al., 1989) but rather base these protocols on the requirements of the current study.

Current fears about the transmissibility of prion diseases place safety at the top of the agenda. Accidental transmission in a research or laboratory setting has now been reported several times (e.g. by Weber et al., 1993), and laboratory staff should be sensitive to this risk. Pathological material should always be regarded as potentially infective. Immunization against hepatitis B is cheap, effective and safe, and should be mandatory.

Dissection technique should be carefully documented and ideally backed up by photographic records. If possible, a trained neuropathologist should be involved at this stage, and in subsequent histopathological evaluation, although it is recognized that this may not always be feasible. Details of the last illness and agonal state, and the interval between death and preservation of brain tissue, should be recorded, since these may have a bearing on the range of methodologies subsequently appropriate. Other collection parameters are likely to be determined by the specific demands of the study; for example, time of death may be of relevance in neuroendocrine work. Finally, and perhaps most importantly, a decision needs to be made between fixation and cryopreservation, and the precise techniques used, as this will determine the types of research methodologies available for future use.

Traditionally, archival material has been stored in formalin, allowing both whole brains and dissected portions to be preserved indefinitely. Concentrations of formalin and other reagents must be standardized and consistent.

Substantial attention has been given to the issue of soft tissue shrinkage that occurs with formalin fixation, suggesting that the final degree of shrinkage depends on the procedure used (e.g. concentration of solution, fixation time, etc.) and the age of the individual from whom the sample was obtained (Uylings, Eden & Hofman, 1986). Newer morphometric techniques now in use, including stereology and image analysis, can take these factors into account with correspondingly improved accuracy of results (Haug, 1986).

Formalin-fixed material allows the use of basic morphometric techniques and standard histological stains such as Nissl, Cresyl Violet, etc. Immunocytochemical studies can also be undertaken, although immunoreactivity may be decreased.

Newer techniques, particularly those such as *in situ* hybridization and radioligand binding (both of homogenized material and in the context of autoradiological studies), which have the potential of providing functional information to complement the structural detail provided by earlier methodologies, require cryopreserved material. The additional problems thus incurred are a price worth paying, although considerable debate continues with regard to minimum time for preservation. There is no generally agreed standard of maximum post-mortem interval, and it has been shown, for example, that some RNAs are stable up to 36 h post-mortem (Barton *et al.*, 1993). It now appears that the availability of very rapidly frozen material, with its attendant dangers of artefactual change, may not be essential.

Administrative considerations

Collection

The perennial problem in establishing a brain banking operation is the lack of suitable material. An NIMH (National Institute of Mental Health) working party recently met to consider approaches to this problem (Wagman, 1992). Among other issues, some of which are touched on above, they reached consensus on the need for the education and training of scientists and clinicians, the investigation of ethical, social and legal obstacles to the use of the Anatomical Gift Act, and the establishment of donor registration programmes, which may be facilitated by liaison with the appropriate health charities. The need for human brain tissue for research purposes is not widely appreciated, the practical aspects of its acquisition may be seen as distasteful, and organ donation for research rather than for transplantation purposes may be held to have lower priority both by the public and by clinicians. Efficient schemes for donor registration must therefore be accompanied by careful liaison with families, health workers, autopsy centres and coroners' courts, if the collection of material is to proceed smoothly and post-mortem interval is to be minimized. This will only be possible with skilled administration and the cultivation of key contacts at a local level.

Dissemination

The dissemination of material to researchers also requires careful organization. Individual brain banks may be able to provide a range of material, with matched control specimens, and Tourtellotte & Berman (1987) have described such a system based on retrieval of computerized and photomicrographic information. Networks of contacts between researchers and brain banks are also beginning to develop, largely on an informal basis, although formal networks, as already developed in other research fields (Clausen *et al.*, 1989), may soon be required. Funding must also be considered, and many brain banking facilities already charge for their services.

Conclusion

Brain banking is of increasing importance in the neurosciences. Although many brain banking facilities are developed in response to specific research needs, in view of the difficulties in obtaining suitable material, maximum flexibility in future scientific applications is to be encouraged. This requires careful documentation of demographic, clinical and technical parameters, attention to the limitations imposed on future research by acquisition and storage protocols, administrative expertise, and the highest ethical standards.

References

American Psychiatric Association (1987). *Diagnostic and statistical manual of mental disorders*. American Psychiatric Association, Washington DC.
Barton, A. J. L., Pearson, R. C. A., Najlerahim, A. & Harrison, P. J. (1993). Pre and post mortem influences on brain RNA. *Journal of Neurochemistry*, **61**, 1–11.
Brahams, D. (1990). Brain banks. *Lancet*, **335**, 282–3.
Clausen, K. P., Grizzle, W. E., Livosi, V. *et al.* (1989). The cooperative human tissue network. *Cancer*, **63**, 1452–9.
Farmer, A. E., McGuffin, P. & Bebbington, P. (1988). The phenomena of schizophrenia. In *Schizophrenia: the major issues* (ed. P. Bebbington & P. McGuffin), pp. 36–50. Heineman, Oxford.
Farmer, A. E., Wessley, S., Castle, D. & McGuffin, P. (1992). Methodological issues in using a polydiagnostic approach to define psychotic illness. *British Journal of Psychiatry*, **161**, 824–30.
Ferrier, I. N. & Perry, E. K. (1992). Post-mortem studies in affective disorder. *Psychological Medicine*, **22**, 835–8.
Haug, H. (1986). History of neuromorphometry. *Journal of Neuroscience Methods*, **18**, 1–17.
Swaab, D. F., Hauw, J.-J., Reynolds, G. P. & Sorbi, S. (1989). Tissue banking and EURAGE. *Journal of the Neurological Sciences*, **93**, 341–3.
Tourtellote, W. W. & Berman, K. (1987). Brain banking. *Encylopedia of Neuroscience*. Vol. 1 (ed. G. Adelman), pp. 156–8. Birkhauser, Boston.
Uylings, H. B. M., Eden, C. G. V. & Hofman, M. A. (1986). Morphometry of size/volume variables and comparison of their bivariate relations in the nervous system under different conditions. *Journal of Neuroscience Methods*, **18**, 19–37.

Wagman, A. M. I. (1992). Report of a workshop on brain tissue acquisition. *Schizophrenia Bulletin*, **18**, 149–52.

Weber, T., Tumani, H., Holdorff, B. *et al*. (1993). Transmission of Creutzfeld–Jakob disease by handling of dura mater. *Lancet*, **341**, 123–4.

Winn, D. M., Reichmann, M. E. & Gunter, E. (1990). Epidemiologic issues in the design and use of biologic specimen banks. *Epidemiologic Reviews*, **12**, 56–70.

2

RNA isolation and analysis

MARK S. PALMER

Types of RNA

RNA analysis is a powerful tool in the determination of tissue- or cell-specific gene expression. While being one step removed from the functional protein product, it is a convenient indicator of the dynamics of gene expression during development or disease, and of gene regulation in response to biological stimuli. In the determination of protein sequence and function following the identification of new partial protein or gene sequences, RNA in the form of complementary DNA (cDNA) is invariably exploited to obtain complete sequences and alternative transcription products, and may be used further for the manipulation of gene expression. Most investigators of gene expression will be concerned with messenger RNA (mRNA). However, in order to interpret the results obtained in practice this discussion will begin with an overview of all RNA types in eukaryotic cells.

The three principal types of cytoplasmic RNA are ribosomal RNA (rRNA), transfer RNA (tRNA) and messenger RNA (mRNA). Each is transcribed in the nucleus as a precursor RNA molecule by one of three RNA polymerases, and then undergoes modification before being transported into the cytoplasm. Three of the four rRNAs (28 S, 5.8 S and 18 S rRNAs) (Noller, 1984) are produced in the nucleolus by RNA polymerase I. A single 13.7 kb (45 S) transcript is produced from clusters of tandemly repeated rDNA genes and is cleaved to produce the three rRNA species 18 S (1.9 kb), 5.8 S (160 bp) and 28 S (5.1 kb) (kb, kilobases; bp, basepairs). There is no known function for the spacer RNA that separates the three products and it is unrelated to intronic sequences of mRNA that are removed by splicing. Cleavage of pre-rRNA does not commence until the complete transcript is synthesized; however, before completion of transcription a number of bases and the ribose groups of specific ribonucleotides are modified by methylation. In the ribosome, 28 S and 5.8 S rRNA associate and together with 5 S rRNA, produced independently, constitute the RNA content of the large (60 S) ribosomal subunit, while 18 S rRNA is associated with the smaller (40 S) ribosomal subunit. rRNA accounts for about 80% of the RNA of a cell and will thus constitute the bulk of total RNA extracted for analysis.

The small RNA molecules, less than 300 bp, including tRNAs and the 5 S (120 bp) rRNA, are synthesized by RNA polymerase III outside the nucleolus region. The rRNA is unique in being synthesized as a functional product requiring no further modification. The tRNAs, which average about 75–80 nucleotides (Holley, 1968) in length and constitute about 15% of total RNA, are synthesized from the multiple copies of the tRNA genes as precursors that require shortening as they mature and are extensively modified by the addition of methyl and isopentyl groups and by the conversion of uridines into pseudouridines. The aminoacylation of tRNAs shows variable kinetics within different brain cells (Vadeboncoeur & Lapointe, 1980). Rat neuronal cells show an initial lag in the synthesis of tRNA^{Glu}, catalysed by high molecular weight complexes of aminoacyl tRNA synthetases not seen in glial cells. The kinetics of formation of tRNA^{Asp} and tRNA^{Val} is linear in both cell types.

mRNA is derived from that class of nuclear RNA referred to as heteronuclear RNA (hnRNA), which term includes all classes of RNA found in the nucleus outside the nucleolar region and transcribed by polymerase II. Nearly all eukaryotic mRNAs are synthesized in a similar manner and are mostly monocystronic. To the 5' cap end of the functional transcription unit (the gene) is a promoter region. The expression of each gene is regulated by the binding of different transcription factors in this promotor region, which ultimately determine whether RNA polymerase II will initiate transcription. The first nucleotide of the primary hnRNA transcript becomes the first nucleotide of the mature mRNA (Dingwall, 1991). When the primary transcript is about 20–30 nucleotides long the initial nucleotide is modified by a 5'–5' linkage to 7-methyl guanylate (m^{7}G), which constitutes the 5' cap structure of mRNA. Transcription continues into a termination region and 3' sequences are removed by endonuclease activity at a site known as the polyadenylation site. The exposed 3' hydroxyl group is then rapidly extended by the addition of 200–250 adenylate residues, which are known as the poly(A) tail (Humphrey & Proudfoot, 1988) (histones are not polyadenylated). The maturing RNA molecule is then further processed by the splicing out of all intervening sequences leaving a contiguous sequence of exons. The mature mRNA that leaves the nucleus contains an open reading frame (ORF), which is directly translated into protein, flanked by 5' and 3' untranslated sequences and bound by the 5' and 3' poly(A) sequences. Translation of the ORF initiates with AUG (methionine) codon and terminates with one of the stop codons (UGA, UAA, UAG). The presence of a poly(A) tail can be exploited in the separation of mRNA from other RNA types.

RNA associated with the expression of mitochondrial genes, including mitochondrial transfer RNAs and ribosomal RNAs, remain within the mitochondria and are not exported to the cytoplasm. Transcription of mitochondrial DNA occurs at just two sites. Transcript I is cleaved to form tRNA^{Phe}, tRNA^{Val}, 12 S and 16 S rRNA, while all the remaining mRNAs and tRNAs are derived from transcript II. There are a few untranslated sequences in human mitochondrial RNAs. The first bases at the 5′ end are usually the AUG (or AUA) initiator codons and the message terminates with a UAA codon, the final As sometimes being part of the added poly(A) tail.

Consideration for handling RNA

Contrary to popular belief RNA is not more unstable than DNA, however, there are important differences in the enzymes that degrade them that have to be borne in mind when handling RNA. DNAase is a fragile enzyme that is easily destroyed by heat, denaturants or physical trauma. However, RNAase is a more robust enzyme, which is difficult to inactivate and which readily renatures if removed from denaturing solution. The handling of RNA is complicated by the ever-present risk of exposure to RNAase and vigorous protocols are required to inactivate and remove the degrading enzyme. Because RNA is a single-stranded molecule and is isolated in lengths of just a few kilobases it is not subject to the same constraints imposed on high molecular weight genomic DNA and is not broken by physical shearing. However, because of the hydroxyl group on the 2′ ribose moiety, the phosphodiester bond between adjacent nucleotides is susceptible to being broken by strong bases. So, while bases such as sodium hydroxide will cause only strand separation of DNA, they will destroy RNAs. This can of course be useful in removing traces of contaminating RNA.

Because of the ever-present problem of RNAase, a number of precautions are usually taken when extracting and handling RNA, and until a laboratory is used to handling RNA routinely a state of paranoid awareness is probably necessary if degradation is to be avoided. It is usual that all laboratory items including glassware, chemicals and, where appropriate, electrophoresis tanks, are reserved exclusively for RNA work (Leibowitz & Young, 1989). Glassware used for storing solutions should first be baked, either at 180 °C for 12 h or at 240 °C for 2 h. In practice, thorough autoclaving is usually found to be adequate, but if degradation remains a persistent problem, return to baking. Chemicals such as sodium chloride or Tris should be poured from new supplies rather than using spatulas, unless these also have been baked. Solutions, which should all be made up with deionized distilled water, are treated by adding diethyl pyrocarbonate (DEPC) to 0.1% to denature RNAase overnight. DEPC is then destroyed by autoclaving. Stir bars should not be used unless they have been baked beforehand. Solutions containing Tris should not be treated with DEPC as Tris causes DEPC to break down, but should be made up with DEPC-treated autoclaved water, and then reautoclaved. (Care should be observed when opening bottles of DEPC, as in the presence of moisture it can decompose to give CO_2, which causes a build-up of pressure in the container.) It is often recommended that fresh gloves are worn when handling or preparing solutions used in RNA work, though this may lead to a certain amount of complacency, and should not be necessary if appropriate care is taken. Sterile plasticware is assumed to be RNAase free but small 1.5 ml tubes and pipette tips, unless supplied sterile, should be autoclaved in small batches. Once opened, a batch should be used immediately, and excess tubes should be used for something else rather than leaving for the next day where dust carrying RNAase could settle on them. A clean working environment is desirable and in many laboratories it may be necessary to ensure that windows are closed to prevent street dust blowing in while working with RNA. First attempts at extracting RNA often prove more successful if performed at weekends or evenings when it is quieter and there are fewer distractions or air currents.

Methods of isolating RNA

There are many protocols available for the isolation of RNA and choosing the appropriate one will depend upon the type of cell or tissue type used, the amount of tissue, which obviously determines the yield, and the use to which the RNA will be put (Maniatis, Fritsch & Sambrook, 1989; Chirgwin *et al.*, 1979). The method of choice will also depend upon whether it is necessary or not to obtain high molecular weight genomic DNA from the same preparation. RNAase is stored within the lysosomes of living cells, but will be released to destroy RNA as soon as a cell is disrupted or dies. If RNA is to be extracted from tissues it must be fresh. Even on ice, extracts have just a few hours before the RNA will begin to degrade. If tissue cannot be processed immediately it should be snap frozen, preferably in liquid nitrogen, and stored frozen at or below $-70\,°C$. RNA can be successfully extracted from frozen tissue weeks later if stored at $-70\,°C$ or even months later if kept in liquid nitrogen, however, because of cell disruption RNA will begin to degrade the moment that the tissue begins to thaw, so never allow frozen tissue to thaw, even on ice. Cell suspensions from tissue culture or blood samples are easily processed but a little more care is required with tissues. Fresh tissues need to be homogenized in lysis buffer after cutting into small pieces. The best way to disperse frozen tissue is to grind it in a pestle under liquid nitrogen. Cool the pestle and mortar first on dry ice, then with liquid nitrogen until it is sufficiently cool to stay liquid without immediately evaporating. The tissue can then be crushed care-fully under liquid nitrogen and ground into a fine powder. This can be added to the lysis solution directly.

The two commonest ways of extracting RNA from the lysis buffer are direct precipitation or separation over a caesium chloride cushion. RNA can be directly precipitated from tissues lysed in 3 M LiCl/6 M urea buffer containing 0.05% SDS (Leibowitz & Young, 1989). Urea serves to denature protein, including RNAase, while LiCl precipitates the RNA (usually overnight at 4 °C). In order to prevent DNA coprecipitation it is necessary to shear the lysed tissue sample in a Polytron homogenizer or equivalent. This method has the disadvantage of not permitting simultaneous isolation of DNA but does give a good yield, and is efficient at extracting high molecular weight RNA species.

For tissues rich in RNAase, the lysis buffer of choice contains guanidium thiocyanate, followed by centrifugation over a caesium chloride cushion in a swing-out rotor (Chirgwin *et al.*, 1979). The density of CsCl is such that the RNA passes through to form a pellet in the bottom of the tube, DNA forms a viscous layer above the cushion and the protein-rich supernatant containing RNAase is above this. Since RNAase is renatureable following dilution of guanidinium thiocyanate, it is necessary to aspirate off the upper layer carefully (retaining the DNA if this is required) and then invert the tube while it still contains CsCl, to pour off the remaining supernatant. The bottom of the tube containing the pelleted RNA is then cut off while still inverted so that the RNA can be physically isolated from the contaminated tube walls. While I have always found this method to give adequate yields of good quality RNA from a variety of tissues and cell lines and rarely have degradation, yields can be improved up to ten fold using Tris/EDTA/Sarkosyl buffers. However, Tris/EDTA/Sarkosyl buffers are less useful when there is a high risk of RNAase presence, such as is found in granulocytes and pancreatic tissues.

After washing and reprecipitation, the yield of RNA can be determined spectrophotometrically on diluted samples at wavelengths of 260 and 280 nm. A clean RNA preparation should have an A_{260}:A_{280} ratio of 2. An $A_{260} = 1$ is equivalent to a concentration of 40 mg ml^{-1}. However, the quality of RNA can only be determined by electrophoresis on formamide gels.

Separation of poly(A)$^+$ RNA

The poly(A) tail can be exploited in the isolation of mRNA because of its complementarity to oligo(dT) (oligonucleotide of 15–20 base pairs composed solely of thymidylate residues) (Aviv & Leder, 1972). Total RNA can be passed over an oligo(dT)–cellulose column in high salt buffer. This stabilises the hybridisation between poly(A) and oligo(dT). The poly(A)$^-$ RNA is eluted in medium salt buffer and, when no more washes off, the mRNA is eluted in low salt buffer. Oligo(dT) columns can be reused a few times, NaOH treatment ensuring elimination of contaminating samples, and often a used column gives a better yield than a new one. Because the amount of RNA recovered (2–5% of total cellular RNA) is quite small, exact quantification is difficult unless directly eluted into clean quartz cuvettes to measure the optical density, although I have never considered committing any of my samples to the spectrophotometer. A reasonably good way is comparative dilution. RNA is often eluted from the oligo(dT) column in 300 μl aliquots and is usually all off in the first 3 ml (from a 0.5 ml column). The elution profile can be determined by spotting 2 μl eluant onto a 1% agarose gel containing 250 μg ml^{-1} ethidium bromide (for convenience this can be poured in a Petri dish and allowed to dry). A fluorescent ring is seen under u.v. illumination, the intensity of which increases with RNA concentration and is a surprisingly sensitive technique for detection of RNA. After RNA-containing aliquots have been pooled and concentrated by precipitation, the concentration can be estimated by dotting dilutions of the material onto the agarose and comparing fluorescence with those of dilutions of total RNA of known concentration determined spectro-photometrically.

A new commercially available method for isolating mRNA in one step from tissue homogenates uses biotin-coupled oligo(dT). The poly(A)$^+$ complex is then bound to avidin-coated magnetic beads, which are removed with a magnet. The non-poly(A)$^+$ RNA is simply washed away. Extraction by this method gives good quality RNA but of low yield and some investigators say that they have difficulty in removing all of the oligo(dT) from their product. As with most processes in molecular biology, the availability of commercial kits for the isolation of RNA will make the procedure more amenable and appealing to researchers from a diverse range of fields.

Analysing RNA

Many of the techniques described below are important in defining the transcriptional unit as isolated from different tissues or cell types. An increasing number of genes, such as the D_2 dopamine receptor gene (Giros *et al.*, 1989) and the β-amyloid precursor protein gene (Tanaka *et al.*, 1988), show differential splicing to produce a number of gene products. Once different forms have been isolated, sequence-specific probes can be used to follow the spatial and temporal regulation of genes and their products. The most elegant and informative method for following the dynamics of RNA expression in the brain during development, disease or in response to medication, is the method of *in situ* hybridization discussed in detail in Chapter 4. However, crude comparisons of levels of RNA expression can more conveniently be performed by Northern or dot blotting of RNA preparations. The problem in any comparative study is quantification and performing the right controls is essential. Changes in expression during development must also take into account changes in cell number and cell size and variation of specific transcripts compared to the total pool of RNA. It is usual in Northern blot analysis to use a probe such as actin mRNA to demonstrate that there is an equal loading of RNA in each lane of the gel. However, while brain actin mRNA is maintained at constant level through most of development and adult life there is a peak of production at day 1 postnatal in the mouse, which declines over the next 15 days to the steady level (Lazarini, Deslys & Dormont, 1991). Glial fibrillary acidic protein mRNA, in contrast, increases in the period of astroglial proliferation during the first weeks of birth and declines until the adult stage during astroglial cell differentiation.

Changes in levels of RNA expression following treatment with drugs or neurotrophic factors must be seen in the context of generalized alteration of rates of transcription and metabolic turnover. Increased levels of mRNA do not always lead to increased levels of protein production. Differential termination of transcription can result in mRNA products of slightly different lengths utilizing different polyadenylation sites, as seen in human oestrogen receptor and glucocorticoid receptor mRNAs (Hollenberg *et al.*, 1985; Green *et al.*, 1986). It is believed that the use of different polyadenylation sites may alter the mRNA stability and result in faster turnover.

Qualitative changes in mRNA expression are less ambiguous. For example, inducing neuronal differentiation in the PC12 cell line with nerve growth factor results in differential splicing of β-amyloid precursors mRNAs, the largest precursor (APP_{770}) being reduced on expression while the shortest (APP_{695}) is increased (Smith, Wion & Brachet, 1991).

An additional difficulty in RNA measurement from tissues is the heterogeneity of cell type present in the sample. While regional variation can be followed, assumptions have to be made about the cell specificity of certain transcripts when individual cell types cannot be teased out. The alteration in expression of glial fibrillary acidic protein (GFAP) or sulphated glycoprotein-2 (SGP-2) mRNAs in response to corticosterone in the hippocampus (Tardy *et al.*, 1984) may be taken as an indication of the astrocyte response to glucocorticoids, but since the production of SGP-2 by neurones has not been excluded, the interpretation of results may be confused (May *et al.*, 1990). Many difficulties of this kind can be resolved by *in situ* hybridization or colocalization by immunoreactivity. Indeed immunohistochemistry may be the only way of accurately determining the consequences of altered gene transcription for the final functional product.

Northern blotting

As with restriction fragments of DNA, RNA can be size fractionated by agarose gel electrophoresis. The RNA can then be blotted onto nitrocellulose or nylon membranes. RNA is usually run in formaldehyde-containing gels in MOPS (morpholinic sulphonic acid) buffer, although RNA extracted with guanidinium thiocyanate may not always give very sharp bands on formaldehyde gels. RNA can be visualized by immersing gels in $250~\mu g\,ml^{-1}$ ethidium bromide for 15 min and destained in water. Ethidium bromide can be added to the RNA solution before loading, however this does not give optimal gel running or transfer conditions. RNA size ladders are commercially available and should be used in preference to DNA size markers as the migration of RNA and DNA on gels is different. Usually size markers are run on a separate lane away from the rest of the RNA and cut off for ethidium bromide staining, thus avoiding staining the whole gel. When total RNA is visualized on formaldehyde gels, the 18 S and 28 S rRNA levels should be clear and bright with the rest of the RNA smeared from about 8 kb down. RNA above 8 kb will be present in less abundance so appears less bright on the gel.

After blotting, RNA filters can be hydridized to DNA or RNA probes, usually in formamide-containing buffer or phosphate buffers. Hybridization in formamide buffers can be performed at lower temperatures (42 °C), which helps to preserve the integrity of the blot and usually gives cleaner results, depending on the gel.

Northern blotting of mRNA can be used to determine the correct size of a transcript (particularly if it is proposed to isolate cDNAs) and to establish whether there is expression of that transcript in individual tissues. When comparing transcription between different tissues it is necessary to use as a control a gene probe such as actin that is expressed at fairly constant copy numbers per cell, in order to ensure that quantitative differences are real and not due to differences in loading the gel or yield of RNA during preparation. The same filter should be used for both probes. RNA bound to nitrocellulose is suitable for multiple use following stripping of probe and, because of the lower temperatures used, the nitrocellulose is less brittle than when used for Southern blots.

cDNA libraries

The term library here implies a large collection of discrete bacterial colonies or phage plaques, each containing copies of a single RNA molecule, reverse transcribed into DNA and subcloned into suitable bacterial or phage vectors. A library can be blotted onto membranes and the filters screened to identify the colony of phage that contains the cDNA of interest. Careful alignment permits the appropriate colony or plaque to be picked from the original plate, which is then grown to give the desired product in quantity.

The first step in constructing a cDNA library is to reverse transcribe mRNA. This is depicted in Figure 2.1. A generalized cDNA library representing all mRNA species can be derived from products primed with oligo(dT). Alternatively, if a partial 3′ sequence is known, transcript-specific enrichment will be achieved using sequence-specific oligonucleotide primers. Reverse transcription yields an RNA:DNA heteroduplex where the DNA is complementary to the RNA sequence. There are two ways of converting this into double-stranded DNA. If the heteroduplex is treated with NaOH and heat, the strands will separate and the RNA is destroyed. The single-stranded cDNA will form a hairpin 'snapback' secondary structure at its 3′ end. This serves as a primer for second-strand synthesis using DNA polymerase. The hairpin loop will contain non base-paired single-stranded DNA that can be cleaved with S1 nuclease. The remaining overlay is blunt-ended with T4 DNA polymerase and subcloned into suitable vectors. (Details of subcloning strategies are beyond the scope of this chapter but include direct blunt end cloning, 3′ oligo(dG) tailing or linker addition to introduce unique restriction sites.) The disadvantage of this technique is that the snapback process will result in cDNAs that are truncated at the 5′ coding end, and probably contain rearrangements. This problem is

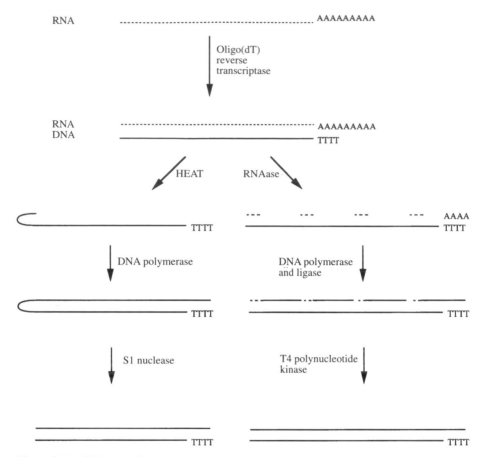

Figure 2.1. cDNA synthesis by two methods. RNA, shown as dashed lines, serves as a template for reverse transcriptase. The resulting DNA:RNA duplex can either be treated with heat to destroy RNA or with RNAase in the presence of DNA polymerase and ligase. The cDNA resulting from heat destruction of RNA automatically snaps back to form a new primer for polymerase. However it causes rearrangements to occur at the 5′ end.

usually avoided by using a second approach that treats the RNA/DNA duplex with RNAase A (an endonuclease) together with DNA polymerase. Partial digestion of the RNA strand retains fragments of RNA that serve as primers for the polymerase. The addition of ligase to the reaction mix ensures that all fragments so formed are linked. The RNA primers are eventually all digested or displaced by DNA polymerase. The product is again polished off at the ends and subcloned. Despite the reduced potential for 5′ rearrangements I have still encountered occasional snapback products using this technique (Palmer *et al.*, 1990) and sequences should be checked for 5′ complementarity using available molecular biology software.

For the isolation of sequences that are more than a few kilobases it may be necessary to use a vector cloning system such as that described by Okayama *et al.* (1987) for the preparation of a cDNA library. This approach uses a single nucleotide tailing strategy to anchor the 3′ cDNA sequences before second-strand synthesis.

One of the limitations in obtaining full length cDNA products, besides degradation of the RNA, is secondary structure formation. Internal complementary sequences can form strongly associated step loop structures that provide an impasse for reverse transcriptase. This may be overcome by briefly warming the RNA solution before proceeding with reverse transcription or by the use of denaturing solvents that are not incompatible with the function of reverse transcriptase. Secondary structure problems may also be encountered with primer extension analysis as described below and in some of the PCR-based approaches to RNA analysis.

A further consideration in the construction of a cDNA library is how large to make it. A message that exists only as 0.01% total mRNA will require at least 100 000 colonies in order to have a reasonable chance of finding at least one copy. Messages more abundant than this can be adequately isolated from libraries prepared in bacterial plasmids; equal or less abundant messages will require λ phage vectors, even if cDNA has been enriched using sequence-specific primers.

A number of cDNA libraries are now commercially available from a range of human and non-human tissues (adult and fetal). These are often suitable for moderately abundant mRNAs of less than 2 kb, but for larger or rarer transcripts are probably best avoided unless by 'personal recommendation'.

Primer extension

In order to identify the true 5′ nucleotide of a transcript, or to resolve differences in splicing at the 5′ end, it is often necessary to use approaches such as primer extension or nuclease protection assays (Calzone, Britten & Davidson, 1987), both of which require some prior sequence or mapping knowledge. For high resolution mapping at the 5′ of a sequence a synthetic oligonucleotide is synthesized complementary to a sequence within about 200 bp of the presumed 5′ terminus. The oligonucleotide is 5′ end labelled by phosphorylation with T4 kinase and $[\gamma^{32}P]ATP$ and used as a primer for reverse transcription of RNA. The samples are then heat denatured and run on urea acrylamide high resolutuion sequencing gels. If the product is run alongside a sequencing reaction from control DNA (such as vector), the exact length of the extended product can be determined to the nearest nucleotide. The size of the products observed may be slightly shorter than the full length, possibly due to the methylation of the first or second nucleotides of the gene transcript. Artefacts may also arise if the priming oligo cross-reacts with other gene transcripts.

In the absence of sufficient sequence information to design synthetic primers, short restriction fragments of the gene, less than 100 bp, can be used and continuously labelled as primer. Single-stranded probes work best but are not absolutely necessary as RNA:DNA duplexes are stronger than DNA:DNA duplexes.

Nuclease protection assay

Nuclease protection assay can be used to give precise information not only about 5′ transcript sites but also the position of introns in genomic sequences. Usually it is used to characterize mRNA with respect to isolated genomic fragments that may have been well characterized by restriction mapping and/or sequencing. In principle, the genomic clone is used as a source of single-stranded continuously or end-labelled DNA or RNA, which is hybridized to mRNA. Only those sequences that are complementary will bind to form duplexes; all excess 3′ or 5′ genomic sequences or introns will remain single stranded. (Or, if partial genomic clones are used, there will be single-stranded mRNA too.) Single-stranded material is then digested with single-strand specific endo- or exonucleases, the remaining double-stranded DNA is size fractionated on high resolution acrylamide gels and the precise location of junctions of complementarity can be determined. Single-stranded DNA probes can be prepared from subcloned genomic sequences using DNA polymerase and suitable primers in the presence of $[\alpha^{32}P]dATP$. End-labelling of restriction fragments can also be used to pin-point unambiguously whether a site lies in the transcribed region or not. A suitable nuclease that will not cleave internal (intronic) sequences is exonuclease VII. Mung bean nuclease and S1 nuclease have endonuclease activity that will not only destroy non-paired regions but may attack regions of low stability such as A:T rich regions. The enzyme chosen will depend on the information required.

RNA probes can be used as an alternative to DNA in a variety of applications. Many available vectors (pUC series or Bluescript, for example) have sites for the initiation of RNA polymerases flanking the subclone insert. These include T3, T7 and SP6 RNA polymerase initiation sites. Vectors can be linearized so that RNA derived from one of these initiation sites will be complementary to the insert DNA and not extend into the vector on the other side. Radiolabelled probes can be prepared by including $[\alpha^{32}P]UTP$ in the polymerase reaction mix. RNA probes are as susceptible to RNAases as other RNA, however directed synthesis can be performed in the presence of RNAase inhibitors such as RNAsin and degradation by RNAase is not normally a problem. (All radioactive nucleic acids will degrade because of radiation damage, and because of the high specific activity of RNA probes, these should be used on the day of preparation.) Because transcripts can be made from either strand of the cloned insert, anti-sense and sense probes can be prepared, which can be used as matched controls for hybridization or protection experiments.

References

Aviv, H. & Leder, P. (1972). Purification of biologically active messenger RNA by chromatography on oligothymidylic acid-cellulose. *Proceedings of the National Academy of Sciences USA*, **69**, 1408–12.

Calzone, F. J., Britten, R. J. & Davidson, E. H. (1987). *Methods in Enzymology*, **152**, 611–32.

Chirgwin, J. M., Przybyla, A. E, MacDonald, R. J. & Rutter, W. J. (1979) Isolation of biologically active ribonucleic acid from sources rich in ribonucleases. *Biochemistry*, **18**, 5294–9.

Dingwall, C. (1991) If the cap fits . . . *Current Biology*, **1**, 65–6.

Giros, B., Solokoff, P., Martres, M. P. *et al.* (1989). Alternative splicing directs the expression of two D_2 dopamine receptor isoforms. *Nature*, **342**, 923–6.

Green, S., Walter, P., Kumar, V. *et al.* (1986). Human oestrogen receptor cDNA: sequence, expression and homology to *v-erb-A*. *Nature*, **320**, 134–9.

Hollenberg, S. M., Weinberger, C., Ong, E. S. *et al.* (1985). Sequence of the human glucocorticoid receptor. *Nature*, **318**, 635–41.

Holley, R. W. (1968). The nucleotide sequence of a nucleic acid. *Scientific American* **214**, 30–9.

Humphrey, T. & Proudfoot, N. J. A. (1988). A beginning to the biochemistry of polyadenylation. *Trends in Genetics*, **4**, 243–5.

Lazarini, F., Deslys, J.-P. & Dormont, D. (1991). Regulation of the glial fibrillary acidic protein, β actin and prion protein mRNAs during brain development in mouse. *Molecular Brain Research*, **10**, 343–6.

Leibowitz, D. & Young, K. (1989). RNA isolation and processing. *Methods in Haematology*, **21**, 37–50.

May, P. C., Lampert-Etchells, M., Johnson, S. A. *et al.* (1990). Dynamics of gene expression for a hippocampal glycoprotein elevated in Alzheimer's disease and in response to experimental lesions in rat. *Neuron*, **5**, 831–9.

Noller, H. F. (1984). Structure of ribosomal RNA. *Annual Review of Biochemistry*, **53**, 119–62.

Okayama, H., Kawaichi, M., Brownstein, M. *et al.* (1987). High efficiency cloning of full length cDNA: construction and screening of cDNA libraries for mammalian cells. *Methods in Enzymology*, **154**, 3–28.

Palmer, M. S., Berta, P., Sinclair, A. H. *et al.* (1990). Comparison of human *ZFY* and *ZFX* transcripts. *Proceedings of the National Academy of Science, USA*, **87**, 1681–5.

Sambrook, J., Fritsch, E. F. & Maniatis, T. (eds.) (1989). *Molecular cloning: a laboratory manual*, edn 2. Cold Spring Harbor, New York.

Smith, C. J., Wion, D. & Brachet, P. (1991). Nerve growth factor-induced differentiation is accompanied by differential splicing of β-amyloid precursor mRNAs in the PC12 cell line. *Molecular Brain Research*, **10**, 351–4.

Tanaka, S., Nakamura, S., Ueda, K. *et al.* (1988). Three types of amyloid protein precursor mRNA in human brain: their differential expression in human brain. *Biochemical and Biophysical Research Communications*, **157**, 472–9.

Tardy, M., Rolland, B., Fages, C. & Caldini, M. (1984). Astroglial cells: glucocorticoid target cells on the brain. *Clinical Neuropharmacology*, **7**, 296–302.

Vadeboncoeur, C. & Lapointe, J. (1980). Slow diffusion of glutamate and ATP–Mg into high molecular weight complexes containing the glutamyl-tRNA synthetase from bovine brain. *European Journal of Biochemistry*, **109**, 581–7.

3

Polymerase chain reaction

MARK S. PALMER

Introduction

Since its introduction in 1985 (Saiki *et al.*, 1985) the polymerase chain reaction, PCR, has revolutionized the way that we are able to perform experiments in molecular biology. The ability to amplify specific sequences from a small amount of starting material, down to a single cell, has added a level of sensitivity not available in any of the conventional techniques such as Southern blotting or *in situ* hybridization. Because it is also very rapid, PCR is often the method of choice in a number of cases even when other options are available. The number of applications to which the PCR can be put means that questions that we could not otherwise have answered can now be easily addressed and new methodologies that promise to enable a wider range of problems to be solved are continuing to be devised (Keeler, 1991). It has often been suggested that the importance of PCR is such that not only will every laboratory performing experiments in molecular biology require a PCR machine but soon every individual in such a laboratory will require one. PCR has now become an important part of many of the biological sciences from immunology to entomology, from forensic science to evolutionary biology, and neurology is no exception.

The principles of the polymerase chain reaction are summarized in Figure 3.1. In general, a double-stranded DNA molecule (which may be derived from RNA by reverse transcription) is heat denatured to yield a single-stranded DNA that can serve as template for DNA polymerase. The primers for the polymerase are synthetic oligonucleotides that bracket a region of a few hundred base pairs of sequence. After the primers have annealed to the template DNA, the polymerase will make copies of the template doubling the amount of starting material. If this procedure of denaturation, annealing and chain elongation is repeated a number of times then there is an exponential increase in the product produced. Because each template produced in the first round is restricted at one end by the initiating primer, the product will be limited to just that material lying between the two oligonucleotides. It is usual to perform the reaction for 30–35 cycles. Theoretically, if there was a 100%

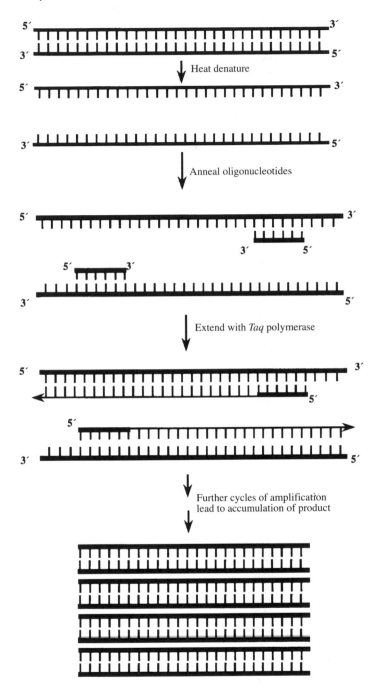

Figure 3.1. The PCR reaction. Double-stranded DNA is denatured at high temperature to give single-stranded DNA. Sequence-specific oligonucleotides are annealed and serve as primers for *Taq* polymerase, which extends the sequence to give new double-stranded molecules. These are again denatured to repeat the process and allow the accumulation of product.

efficiency, each starting molecule would give rise to over 10^9 molecules after 30 cycles. After 30–35 cycles there is sufficient product in the PCR reaction for a small amount of it to be easily visualized on ethidium bromide stained agarose gels, and all products should be of the same length. The product can then be treated as any other DNA product and be subcloned, sequenced, digested, used as hybridization probe or as target for other probes as required. However, the very sensitivity of the reaction introduces its own problems, namely the amplification of contaminating sequences, and the amplification of non-specific sequences by the early cross-hybridization of primers to other sequences, which then enter the cycle with exact oligonucleotide complementary ends.

The purpose of this chapter is to describe many of the applications to which PCR can be put, explaining the sort of problems that may arise with each application and how they may be overcome.

The general procedure for PCR amplification

Despite the widespread use of PCR, our understanding of what goes on in the reaction tube is still surprisingly incomplete. As a consequence, the conditions for each new reaction essentially have to be determined anew empirically. Many PCR artefacts generated cannot easily be explained and the only solution is to alter the parameters until the quality of the product improves. As a general rule, it is sufficient to start from a standard reaction condition and alter the parameters to be either more or less stringent depending upon whether there are too many artefacts or too little product of any kind. The following is a guide to the standard conditions and to which parameters can be altered to optimize the reaction (Innis & Gelfand, 1990).

The standard conditions (usually a 100 μl reaction volume) use a buffer of 50 mM KCl, 20 mM Tris-HCl (pH 8.3, 40 °C) 0.02% gelatin and $MgCl_2$ at 1.5 mM. The reaction is sensitive to the concentration of $MgCl_2$ and this is one of the factors that can be varied to improve the reaction. dNTPs are added to the buffer at a final concentration of 200 μM of each dNTP. Of each oligonucleotide primer, 25 pmol is used, together with 2.5 units of *Taq* polymerase. *Taq* polymerase is a thermostable DNA polymerase from the bacterium *Thermus aquaticus*, originally marketed by Perkin Elmer Cetus and now available from this company as a recombinant gene product *amplitaq* (Saiki & Gelfand, 1989). A number of new polymerases are being developed by other companies from bacteria living at high temperatures in order to exploit their individual characteristics for use in the PCR reaction. Vent (a trademark of New England Biolabs) is derived from *Thermococcus litoralis* and Stratagene's *Pfu* from *Pyrococcus furiosus*. The new generation enzymes are being chosen with a view to their thermostability and their fidelity of DNA synthesis.

To this reaction is added the template DNA at an optimum of 10^5–10^6 template molecules per reaction. One microgram of human genomic DNA equals 3×10^5 target molecules, though with many genes it is possible to go down to 10 ng genomic DNA and still obtain sufficient amplification after 35 cycles. Before the reaction is initiated, the sample is overlayered with mineral oil to avoid evaporation. Automated thermal cyclers ('PCR machines') now allow the construction of linked thermal programmes with a variety of ramp rates and extension parameters. Although this often adds too much complexity for most applications, it is of particular use to be able to initiate the reaction with a single denaturation stage of 94 °C for 5 min before starting the cyclic series. This is important for genomic DNA, which requires longer denaturation times than PCR products in order to overcome its greater thermal stability particularly in G + C-rich regions of the genome. This is followed by the 30–35 cycles of the following temperature profile:

> denaturation: 94 °C, 30 s
> primer annealing: T_m °C 30 s, where T_m is the theoretical melting temperature T_M of the primers plus 5 °C
> primer extension: 72 °C, 45 s

Cycling is followed by a final extension at 72 °C for 5 min. The T_m is determined from the Wallace rule $\{T_M = 2(A + T) + 4(G + C)\}$ (Wallace *et al.*, 1979). In practice most oligonucleotides for PCR will give a T_m of above 50 °C, and in any case should not be annealed above 60 °C. The theoretical melting temperature should be used only as a rough guide as PCR conditions are different from those under which the Wallace rule holds. However, it serves as a useful starting point. The products of a PCR reaction are analysed by running out 10 μl of product on an agarose gel containing ethidium bromide, the agarose concentration depending on the size of the expected product. If there are a number of bands in addition to that which is expected then it will most likely be necessary to increase the temperature of the annealing stage of the reaction to reduce non-specific primer annealing. Conversely, little or no product indicates that a lower temperature should be used.

Parameters affecting PCR reactions

As well as adjusting the temperature of the reaction there are a number of other factors that can be altered to improve the PCR reaction. Some primers are sensitive to the concentration of $MgCl_2$ in the reaction mix. The standard mix contains $MgCl_2$ at 1.5 mM. A titration should be performed from 0.5 mM to 4 mM in 0.5 mM increments and from 4 mM to 10 mM in 1 mM increments to cover the range effectively. Most primers should work well in the 1.5 mM range but occasionally they will give bands only in the highest concentrations. An important factor affecting the efficiency of the PCR reaction is the stability of the template DNA. This is particularly important when using genomic DNA as G + C-rich regions close to the site of amplification could prevent the initial denaturation stage or reassociate rapidly before primers have had an opportunity to anneal. This may be overcome by adding a solvent to the reaction such as

DMSO (dimethyl sulphoxide), formamide or glycerol. For example, 5% (v/v) DMSO is necessary to get amplification of the prion protein gene open reading frame with most primers and improves the specificity of amplification with others. Solvents can be tried at 1%, 5% and 10% concentrations, though they ought not to be required routinely as many primers are inhibited by their addition, or at best it makes no difference.

The concentration of dNTPs also seems to affect some reactions and may be reduced in some reactions to reduce non-specific amplifications. Theoretically, 20 μm of each dNTP is sufficient to synthesize 2.6 μg DNA or 10 pmol of a 400 bp fragment, though allele-specific amplification of *ras* point mutations have been amplified using as little as 2 μm of each dNTP (Ehlen & Dubeau, 1989). Lower dNTP concentrations will probably require less $MgCl_2$ and this should be reduced as well.

Enzyme concentration is another factor that may affect the reaction; 2.5 units of polymerase is usually used in a 100 μl reaction; however, it is worth titrating this down to a tenth of the amount as the enzyme is very stable and very fast (incorporating 60 nucleotides per second) and adequate product may be produced at 0.5 units per 100 μl reaction. Too little enzyme will stop the accumulation of large quantities of product because of its dilution with respect to template, so particularly with longer fragments the enzyme concentration should not be taken too low. Titrating the enzyme for a reaction that is to be used routinely could save a lot of money.

The quality and concentration of template DNA will cause variation between reactions. Inhibitors remaining from the purification of DNA (such as poly-ethylene glycol, PEG) will cause problems and persistently difficult DNA preparations should be cleaned up with fresh phenol/chloroform and repreci-pitated. The DNA should also be titred, as the effective concentration of template depends upon accessibility of the target sequence as much as absolute concentrations. Secondary structure formations in single-stranded DNA may make some sequences less efficient than others, while genomic effects may make some sequences more accessible than others. Prion protein gene amplifi-cation requires 1 μg genomic DNA (even in the presence of DMSO), while amyloid precursor protein exons require only 20 ng of DNA.

Preparation of genomic DNA for PCR

DNA can be extracted for PCR by general protocols such as those that would be used to extract DNA for Southern blot analysis. Although it is particularly important to ensure that there is no cross-contamination of samples, it is not necessary to extract large quantities of DNA. For some applications, such as amplification from blood, it is not necessary to extract DNA and whole cells can be used instead (Mercier *et al.*, 1990). It has been found that 2 μl of blood added directly to the PCR reaction can liberate sufficient DNA for PCR by subjecting the reaction to three or four cycles of high temperature denaturation and cooling before proceeding with the amplification cycles. This obviously has great advantages for rapidly screening large numbers of patients from small blood samples. It is important not to use too much sample as the cellular debris will inhibit the reaction.

Extraction of DNA from formalin-fixed or paraffin-embedded samples is possible but is more difficult and the yield not only unpredictable but of poor quality (Greer, Lund & Manos, 1991). The recovery of DNA from fixed tissues depends on the length of time between removal and fixation, the duration of fixation and, for paraffin-embedded sections, the length of time in the blocks. Formalin-fixed brain can be digested by extensive proteinase-K treatment to release DNA. However, the DNA is fragmented and of low yield. In some cases the extraction can be improved by washing fixed tissue in phosphate-buffered saline before extraction. Paraffin-embedded sections require xylene or other solvents to remove the paraffin before proteinase K digestion of the cellular material.

Amplification of RNA

Before RNA can be amplified it needs to be converted into DNA by reverse transcription. Reverse transcription can be performed using either oligo(dT) as a primer, or by using a three prime sequence specific to the transcript of interest (Figure 3.2). The advantage of using transcript-specific primers is the initial enrichment of target sequences and the reduction in non-specific hybridization that follows. RNA can be extracted by any of the methods described in Chapter 2; however, it is not uncommon for RNA preparations to contain small amounts of contaminating DNA. This is particularly inconvenient for PCR because the amplified DNA signal may be as strong as the RNA signal. To try and remove DNA the RNA preparation can be treated with RNAase-free DNAase before reverse transcription. Even this procedure, however, may not completely eradicate the problem. It is therefore necessary, where possible, to choose oligonucleotide primers that span an intron and would not normally amplify genomic sequences or at least amplify different sizes from genomic DNA than from RNA. This does require that some information concerning the genomic organization of the gene sequence is available. In the absence of suitable sites or information, control experiments will have to be performed, treating the RNA with RNAase before reverse transcription and comparing the signal produced with samples containing RNA.

PCR applications

Mutation analysis

The PCR can be used to screen patients for mutations in genes, either as part of a routine analysis for known mutations or for the identification of new

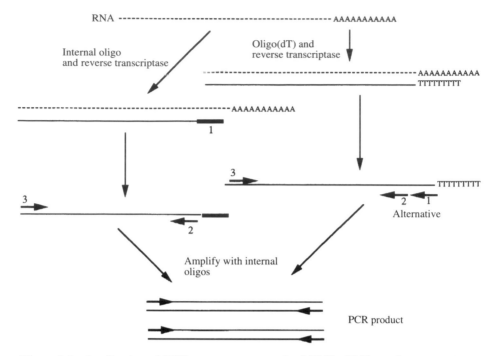

Figure 3.2. Application of PCR to reverse transcribed RNA. RNA can be reverse-transcribed using either oligo(dT) or internal sequence-specific oligonucleotides. PCR uses oligonucleotides that were not used for the reverse transcription process.

mutations (Goate *et al.*, 1991; Palmer *et al.*, 1991). This can be applied to specific diagnostic purposes or for original research. Mutations may either be of the type that alter the size of amplified products (insertions or deletions), or that alter the sequence at specific sites (point mutations or frame shifts). These may be conventionally detected by alterations in restriction fragment visualized by Southern blotting and hybridization. Insertions or deletions within amplified sequences can easily be detected by the alteration in band size on agarose gels. However, it is important to realize that in some cases two alleles that differ in size between two points will not amplify equally. It is well recognized that in the prion protein gene, insertions of sequences in a repetitive region of the gene will give products 144 bp or more larger than normal but that these sequences amplify less efficiently with most primers. It may therefore be possible to miss insertions in a heterozygote unless primers are chosen to optimize amplification first. For small deletions or insertions it may be necessary to choose primers that amplify only short sequences in order to be able to distinguish the products on agarose gels.

Point mutations within amplified products can be detected in a number of ways. Where the mutation causes an alteration in restriction site the sample can simply be digested and products run on a gel. As most people will be heterozygous for sequence variations looked for in this way it is important to be able to resolve the differences in band size in a mixed sample. Most mutations will not give rise to convenient restriction enzyme site differences. Single point differences can then be detected by allele-specific oligonucleotide hybridization (Figure 3.3). The PCR product is transferred to nylon or nitrocellulose filters in a vacuum manifold. Synthetic oligonucleotides of about 15 bp are prepared, which are identical to the normal sequence or to the mutation. The altered base should lie in the middle of the sequence. Duplicate filters can be hybridized to ^{32}P end-labelled oligonucleotides of either sequence. Filters are washed in a solution containing 3 M TEMAC (tetramethylammonium chloride) at a suitable temperature determined empirically. TEMAC removes the difference seen in hybridization temperatures between oligonucleotides of the same length but different nucleotide composition (Wood *et al.*, 1985). At an appropriate temperature, the labelled wild-type oligonucleotide will hybridize only to wild-type sequences while the mutant oligonucleotide will hybridize only to mutant sequences. Hybridization is determined by autoradiography, heterozygotes showing hybridization to both oligonucleotides and homozygotes to one or the other.

New mutations can be detected by the use of denaturing gradient gel

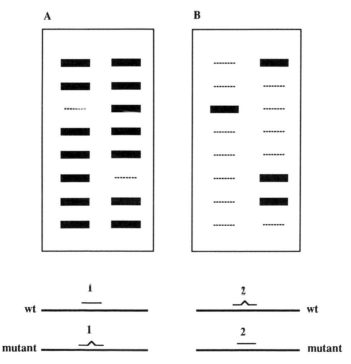

Figure 3.3. Principle of allele-specific oligonucleotide hybridization to detect point mutations. (A) and (B) are duplicate filters containing PCR-amplified material from 16 individuals. These are hybridized to ^{32}P end-labelled oligos that are either identical to the wild type (wt) sequence (oligo 1 hybridized to filter A) or to the point mutation (oligo 2 hybridized to filter B). On these filters there are 12 samples homozygous for wild type, two homozygous for the mutation and two heterozygotes.

electrophoresis (DGGE) or by single-strand conformational polymorphism (SSCP) analysis (Hayashi, 1991). Both procedures rely on the observation that DNA strands with different sequences have different internal melting characteristics and can form different secondary structures. In DGGE an acrylamide gel containing an increasing concentration of denaturants such as urea and formamide is run at a constant high temperature. The denaturing gradient is equivalent to raising the temperature as the product migrates down the gel. As domains within the sequence melt, the DNA is retarded. Provided that mutations do not lie in the last domain to melt, the differences in melting temperature caused by the mutation will alter the time at which the mutant domain melts and cause aberrant retardation. This results in the separated strands from wild type and mutant sequences having different mobilities, which can be detected by ethidium bromide staining of the acrylamide gel. Since this discriminates on the basis of melting characteristics and not band size, it is necessary to perform a number of control runs to optimize the denaturing gradient. For sequences in which the mutation does not lie in the last melting domain, an artificial domain can be created by designing oligonucleotide primers continuing a G + C-rich sequence as a linker. This method of mutation analysis has been reported to give a very high level of detection of novel mutations.

SSCP

This is a much simpler procedure but has a less good detection rate and many mutations cannot be picked up by this method. For SSCP, PCR is performed with ^{32}P end-labelled oligonucleotides or by incorporating radionucleotides into the reaction. Reaction products are run on thin acrylamide gels containing glycerol. Differences in secondary structure between sequences causes differences in migration rate. This method works best with sequences of up to 300 bp but larger sequences can be analysed by first digesting with appropriate restriction enzymes.

Nested PCR

For certain applications the usual 35 cycles of amplification are not sufficient to give visible bands on an agarose gel, although there may be product present. One way to overcome this is to blot gels containing PCR products and to hybridize with appropriate probes. Radiohybridizations of this sort are very sensitive to small amounts of DNA on the filter. However, an alternative is simply to PCR for longer. If the repeated or extended PCR is performed with the same oligonucleotide primers this can lead to a number of problems. Non-specific hybridization to primers at any stage will lead to trace products that are primed with the PCR oligonucleotides. As these contaminants are further amplified they will increase the background. The specificity of amplification can be maintained by choosing a second set of primers slightly internal to the first two which are again specific for the sequence being amplified. Such oligonucleotides are called nested primers and they ensure that in a second round of 35 cycles of PCR amplification only the correctly amplified product during the first round of PCR contributes to product in the second round. The disadvantage of performing nested PCR is that contaminating sequences of the correct sequence may become amplified to a level in excess of the actual target material. For example, DNA extracted from small numbers of cells or single cells may become contaminated by material originating from the operator, such as skin fragments. The DNA may therefore include a significant proportion of DNA from the incorrect source, which will amplify up in the same manner as the correct DNA and contribute to the result. Such contamination would give completely false data. It is therefore necessary to be particularly careful at all stages when performing nested PCR reactions.

Probe preparation

PCR reactions can be performed on any sequence to generate specific probes. For example, cloned cDNA sequences that do not have convenient internal restriction sites can nevertheless be used to prepare exon-specific probes by PCR. A general laboratory method for isolating probes from cloned stocks without having to grow up large quantities of plasmid is to use the vector sequence flanking the insert to amplify insert. If the PCR reaction is performed in the presence of radionucleotides then labelled probe can be rapidly prepared.

Subcloning

There are many ways of subcloning PCR products, but they appear to subclone less efficiently than DNA derived from other sources. Primers can be designed to include unique restriction sites in a linker sequence that can be cut to incorporate the product directly. Alternatively, the product can be blunt-end subcloned into suitable vectors. The primers used for PCR will not normally contain a 5' phosphate group and T4 DNA kinase will have to be used to add one. It is also advisable to use the Klenow fragment of DNA polymerase in order to 'polish' the ends and ensure that they are properly blunted. It is now known that *Taq* polymerase adds an extra adenosine residue to the end of each newly synthesized chain, resulting in a 3' overhang of a single A residue. The enzyme also appears to bind quite tightly to the ends of the double-stranded product and may interfere with enzyme activity at that end of the product. The polymerase association with the product can be overcome by treating with proteinase-K. This should increase the effective concentration of available ends for subcloning. The A overhang can also be exploited by using vectors with a T overhang (Marchuk *et al.*, 1991). Such a vector can be prepared by cutting pUC or Bluescript, for example with a blunt end cutter, and putting the cut vector in a PCR reaction containing just dTTP as nucleotide and setting for a fixed temperature for a couple of hours. The polymerase, in the absence of dATP, will add an additional T to the cut vector. This so called T-vector can be used to subclone the A-tailed PCR product directly without the need to treat with any enzyme (though again proteinase-K may increase the yield).

Sequencing PCR products

Once PCR products have been subcloned they can be sequenced as other sequences, either as double-stranded plasmids or extracted as single-stranded DNA. Although sequencing subcloned products is often easier than the direct methods described below, there are artefacts of PCR reactions that may arise and which have to be taken into account when interpreting sequence. The first is polymerase fidelity. There are varying reports as to the error rate for *Taq* polymerase, but it does depend on the reaction conditions. In particular, high concentrations of dNTPs and $MgCl_2$ are known to increase the error rate and can even be exploited to produce random mutations under controlled conditions. The cumulative error from a number of experiments is probably less than 1 in 10^5 and the mutation rate about 5×10^{-6} per nucleotide incorporating per cycle over 25 cycles using 200 mM dNTPs and 1.5 mM $MgCl_2$. However, when sequencing reveals new mutations it is essential that there is confirmation from a second clone, preferably from an independent PCR subcloning, in order to eliminate the possibility of the mutation being a PCR error.

An additional error in subcloned PCR reactions is the occurrence of so-called shuffle clones. If during the copying of DNA templates the polymerase does not continue to completion, partial products are produced, which can themselves act as primers for the next round of the reaction. However, if this primer associates with template from the other allele (assuming amplification from heterozygous genomic DNA), it will give rise to an effective crossover event in which the partial product from an allele becomes incorporated into the product of the other allele. In that way a polymorphic marker that is being used to detect both alleles in subcloned products may have become removed from a linked mutation and both alleles sequence as though there were no mutations. So again, the absence of mutations in subcloned material needs to be checked by additional sequencing.

One way around these difficulties is to sequence PCR products directly without subcloning so as to produce an average sequence. Different allelic sequences will appear together in the same tracks of the sequencing gel, so this procedure is not suitable for highly polymorphic genes. Direct sequencing requires that the PCR product is first cleaned up by gel exclusion chromatography or membrane filtration and that an oligonucleotide other than that used for PCR is used as the sequencing oligonucleotide. Better results are obtained if the oligo is ^{32}P end-labelled as the products are more specific than those obtained by incorporation of ^{35}S during synthesis. Single-stranded DNA can be generated from a PCR reaction by starting with 100:1 or 50:1 ratio of the oligonucleotides. Initially, double-stranded product is generated in the usual way. As one of the oligonucleotides is depleted so only the remaining primer can be used to initiate synthesis. There is thus a linear increase in the production of DNA from one strand, which produces, after about 35 cycles, DNA of sufficient quantity for sequencing. This is called asymmetric PCR.

Rapid amplification of cDNA ends (RACE)

Chapter 2 describes how the 5′ of a transcribed sequence can be determined by primer extension or by nuclease protection assay. An alternative method using PCR can be adapted to find the 5′ or 3′ end of a sequence, provided that internal sequence is known (Frohman, Dush & Martin, 1988). Reverse transcribed RNA (using either oligonucleotide dT or preferably an internal oligonucleotide primer) is 3′ extended with dGTP using terminal deoxynucleotide transferase (Figure 3.4). A primer containing a unique sequence and a string of Cs is used as the primer for this end (the 5′ end of the coding sequence), together with an internal oligonucleotide that is different from that used for reverse transcription for the 3′ end. It is important not to amplify with the same oligonucleotide as that used for reverse transcription, because of the number of additional molecules that will have been transcribed by non-specific interaction with the primer. 3′ RACE is similarly performed using a T-rich

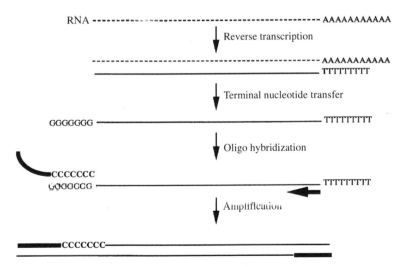

Figure 3.4. Rapid amplification of cDNA ends. Here the 5′ end is amplified by extending the 3′ end of complementary DNA, prepared by reverse transcription, with terminal deoxynucleotide transferase and dGTP. The primer that hybridizes to this G tail contains a linker sequence that helps to anchor the PCR reaction and a tail of Cs. The 3′ end can be similarly amplified using a T-rich oligo linker that hybridizes to the poly(A) tail.

oligonucleotide for the 3′ end and an internal oligonucleotide for the 5′ end. The reaction generally works best for sequences close to the ends and 200 bp is probably optimal for this sort of amplification.

Quantitative PCR

Because of its ability to detect nucleic acids present in low amounts, PCR has been used for the detection of low abundance RNAs from a variety of sources. It has been possible to show a low level of expression of many transcripts in tissues not previously known to demonstrate expression (Chelly *et al.*, 1988). However, because of the amplificatory nature of PCR, it is clear that in some cases amplification corresponds to a few starting molecules amongst many hundreds of cells, rather than a low level of expression within each cell. It is therefore essential for comparative purposes to have some means of quantifying the levels of RNA detected by PCR and a number of methods are now available (Gilliland, Perrin & Bunn, 1990; Wang & Mark, 1990). Quantitation usually requires that a template of known concentration is amplified at the same time as the target RNA by the same primers. The products of amplification need to be distinguishable on agarose gels, either by size or following digestion. The problem of controls of different size is ensuring that different transcripts are amplified at the same rate and that there is not preferential expression of one or other. A cDNA product can be manipulated to contain a new internal restriction site. The cDNA prepared as either double- or single-stranded DNA can be quantitated on a spectrophotometer and then prepared in a dilution ranging from 10 ng to 1 fg. The dilution is made in a large volume (1 ml) so that the same solution can be used for multiple experiments without variation. The diluted material is then added to samples of the reverse transcribed RNA before amplification. All samples will contain the same amount of correct reverse transcribed RNA and a range of concentrations of the mutant cDNA. The products are digested with the enzyme specific for the mutant sequence and compared on agarose gels. Where the intensity of the two bands is equivalent then the concentration of starting reverse transcribed RNA equals the added cDNA. A similar approach is to express RNA from a vector containing the target sequence including the sites for PCR priming. The RNA produced, for example, by T7 RNA polymerase can again be measured in a spectrophotometer and added to the extracted RNA, this time before reverse transcription. PCR is performed with one of the primers end-labelled, and radioactivity in each band product from a range of dilutions plotted on a logarithmic graph such that the mass of starting RNA can be compared with the number of molecules of competing RNA.

It is important for quantification that the PCR is still in the linear phase of reaction when products are compared, in other words that the reaction has not reached a plateau for either template, as then the product concentrations cannot be compared.

Ligase chain reaction (LCR)

A variant on the polymerase chain reaction is a procedure that uses thermostable ligases in a reaction that can be used to discriminate single base differences (Barany, 1991). Allele-specific LCR uses four oligonucleotides, two pairs adjacent to each other and complementary to opposite strands of DNA template (Figure 3.5). The ligase will join adjacent pairs on each strand if they are exactly complementary to the template at their junction. They will in turn, as ligated products, act as substrate for the second round of LCR and so on for a number of cycles. Eventually, product of a single band size is synthesized, which can be detected on gels. If there is a base mismatch at either of the ends to be joined then there will be no ligation and no product. By choosing oligonucleotides of slightly varying lengths to distinguish products amplified in the presence of a mutation from those produced in the absence, it is possible to screen for heterozygotic presence of DNA targets such as haemoglobin variants.

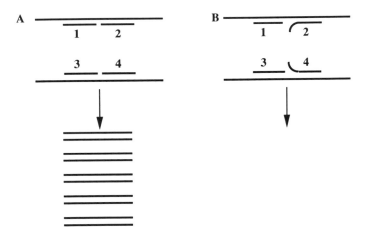

Figure 3.5. Ligase chain reaction. A and B are different alleles of the same gene differing by a single base pair. Oligos 1, 2, 3 and 4 hybridize to sites that flank the base difference and require complete identity for annealing. Oligos 2 and 4 cannot hybridize to the sequence B because they mismatch at the last nucleotide. In the presence of Ligase the oligo pairs 1 and 2 or 3 and 4 ligate when associated with sequence A but cannot ligate on sequence B because of the lack of binding to the template. As the reaction is repeated, more template accumulates from sequence A but none from B. This technique can be used to screen for mutations in an individual, in a single reaction, by the inclusion of a second set of oligos of slightly different lengths, which ligate on sequence B but not on sequence A. If the products are run on agarose or acrylamide gels the presence of both sequences would be indicated by the presence of both size products.

Recombinant PCR

PCR primers will anneal to the starting template at the correct temperature even if there are sequence differences between primer and template (Higuchi, Krummel & Saiki, 1988). These differences may be as small as point mutations or include small insertions. Product generated with such primers will faithfully include the mutation, which can be exploited to generate site-mutated products for experimental purposes. Primers can be designed to include a number of linker sequences. If these are complementary to other sequences from vectors or, for example, the promoters of other genes then PCR products can be generated from simultaneous reactions that serve as primer/templates for each other and generate fused products.

References

Barany, F. (1991) Genetic disease detection and DNA amplification using cloned thermostable ligase. *Proceedings of the National Academy of Sciences, USA*, **88**, 189–93.

Chelly, J., Kaplan, J.-C., Maire, P. *et al*. (1988). Transcription of the dystrophin gene in human muscle and non-muscle tissues. *Nature*, **333**, 858–60.

Ehlen, T. & Dubeau, L. (1989). Detection of *ras* point mutations by polymerase chain reaction using mutation specific, inosine-containing oligonucleotide primers. *Biochemical and Biophysical Research Communications*, **160**, 441–7.

Frohman, M. A., Dush, M. K. & Martin, G. R. (1988). Rapid production of full-length cDNAs from rare transcripts: amplification using a single gene-specific oligonucleotide primer. *Proceedings of the National Academy of Sciences, USA*, **85**, 8998–9002.

Gilliland, G., Perrin, S. & Bunn, H. F. (1990). Competitive PCR for quantitation of mRNA. In *PCR protocols: a guide to methods and applications* (ed. M. A. Innis, D. H. Gelfand, J. J. Sninsky & T. J. White), pp. 60–9. Academic Press, San Diego.

Goate, A., Chartier-Harlin, M.-C., Mullan, M. *et al*. (1991). Segregation of a missense mutation in the amyloid gene with familial Alzheimers disease. *Nature*, **349**, 704–6.

Greer, C. E., Lund, J. K. & Manos, M. M. (1991). PCR amplification from paraffin embedded tissues: recommendations for long-term storage and prospective studies. *PCR Methods and Applications*, **1**, 46–50.

Hayashi, K. (1991). PCR-SSCP: A simple and sensitive method for detection of mutations in the genomic DNA. *PCR Methods and Applications*, **1** 34–8.

Higuchi, R., Krummel, B. & Saiki, R. K. (1988). A general method of *in vitro* preparation and specific mutagenesis of DNA fragments: study of protein and DNA interactions. *Nucleic Acids Research*, **16**, 7351–67.

Innis, M. A. & Gelfand, D. H. (1990). Optimization of PCR. In *PCR protocols: a guide to methods and applications* (ed. M. A. Innis, D. H. Gelfand, J. J. Sninsky & T. J. White), pp. 3–13. Academic Press, San Diego.

Keeler, R. (1991). Uses for PCR are multiplying in gene-related research. *R & D Magazine*, **33**, 30–40.

Marchuk, D., Drumm, M., Saulino, A. & Collins, S. (1991). Construction of T-vectors, a rapid and general system for direct cloning of unmodified PCR products. *Nucleic Acids Research*, **19**, 1154.

Mercier, B., Gaucher, C., Feugeas, O. & Mazurier, C. (1990). Direct PCR from whole blood, without DNA extraction. *Nucleic Acids Research*, **18**, 5908.

Palmer, M. S., Dryden, A. J., Hughes, J. T. & Collinge, J. (1991). Homozygous prion protein genotype predisposes to sporadic Creutzfeldt–Jacob disease. *Nature*, **352**, 340–2.

Saiki, R. K. & Gelfand, D. H. (1989). Introducing AmpliTaq DNA polymerase. *Amplifications*, 4–6.

Saiki, R. K., Scharf, S., Faloona, F. *et al*. (1985). Enzymatic amplification of β-globin genomic sequences and restriction site analysis for diagnosis of sickle cell anemia. *Science*, **230**, 1350–4.

Wallace, R. B., Shaffer, J., Murphy, R. F. *et al*. (1979). Hybridization of synthetic oligodeoxyribonucleotides to phi chi 174 DNA: the effect of single base pair mismatch. *Nucleic Acids Research*, **6**, 3543.

Wang, A. M. & Mark, D. F. (1990). Quantitative PCR. In *PCR protocols: a guide to methods and applications* (ed. M. A. Innis, D. H. Gelfand, J. J. Sninsky & T. J. White), pp. 70–4. Academic Press, San Diego.

Wood, W. I., Gitschier, J., Lasky, L. A. & Lawn, R. M. (1985). Base composition-independent hybridisation in tetramethylammonium chloride: A method for oligonucleotide screening of highly complex gene libraries. *Proceedings of the National Academy of Sciences, USA*, **82** 1585–8.

4

Principles and practice of *in situ* hybridization histochemistry in neuropsychiatric research

PAUL J. HARRISON
and R. CARL A. PEARSON

Introduction

The advent of molecular genetics has provided a new avenue by which to investigate the aetiopathogenesis of neuropsychiatric disorders. Through strategies of linkage analysis and gene sequencing, potential disease loci and causative mutations can be identified, an approach which has already paid dividends in the case of Alzheimer's disease (AD) (Harrison, 1993). Such methods complement and extend the pre-existing investigations into the structural pathology and neurochemical changes occurring in a disorder; for example, in AD, these latter approaches have, respectively, identified the composition of neurofibrillary tangles and the presence of cholinergic deficits.

Linking these aspects of disease aetiopathogenesis is gene expression, the term given to the many processes and mechanisms by which the information contained in the genome is realized in the precise spatial and temporal production of proteins. For example, its study can help explain how a candidate gene may cause a disorder by virtue of its pattern of expression and its alteration in disease, thereby relating a genetic abnormality to a pathological phenotype. Moreover, this principle need not be restricted to candidate genes, since a generalized or gene-specific alteration in some aspect of gene expression, whether qualitative or quantitative in nature, may underlie multiple pathological or biochemical features of a disorder.

Given the importance of gene expression in the overall understanding of the molecular basis of disease, a variety of techniques are available for its investigation. Most techniques for evaluating cerebral gene expression in a disease rely on measuring some facet of messenger RNA (mRNA), since mRNA is the main intermediate between a gene and its protein product; it is formed by the process of transcription and gives rise to the encoded peptide by translation and protein synthesis. Essentially, there are four parameters of mRNA that can be determined: its presence, its abundance, its intactness (integrity), and its biological activity (its ability to serve as a template for protein synthesis). Each of these parameters may be measured for mRNA as a whole, providing an indicator of overall gene expression, or for specific mRNAs, providing information about the expression of a particular gene. It should be noted that the present emphasis upon RNA as the main marker of gene expression does not imply that other aspects of the process are unimportant – indeed it is essential to investigate many other parameters (e.g. Crapper McLachlan & Lewis, 1985) – but reflects the fact that RNA is the most accessible component of gene expression in the present context.

Techniques for detecting an individual mRNA rely on the principle of nucleic acid hybridization, whereby a single strand of DNA or RNA (a 'probe') will, under suitable conditions, bind ('hybridize') to its complementary strand (in this situation, an mRNA of interest) by nucleotide base pairing. By prior labelling of the probe, the localization of hybridization, and thus of the mRNA in question, can be determined. Hybridization methodologies of this kind may be carried out on filters (Northern blots) or in solution. A further hybridization methodology, based on identical principles, is *in situ* hybridization histochemistry (ISHH). ISHH allows the detection of mRNA present within tissue sections, as opposed to the above techniques, which require the prior extraction of RNA from homogenized tissue.

The unique ability to study mRNAs without destroying tissue structure gives ISHH particular roles in the study of brain gene expression in health and disease. These are reviewed in the first part of this chapter, together with a summary of the existing data resulting from the application of ISHH to neuropsychiatric disorders; the second part discusses the problems associated with the use of human brain tissue for ISHH and related techniques, and the practical factors to be considered when setting up ISHH in this field. Throughout, emphasis is given to research using human material, since in the absence of satisfactory animal models of neuropsychiatric diseases this remains the only direct means of investigation, and its particular problems have sometimes been neglected. ISHH also has extensive applications in other areas of research, for which a somewhat different set of conceptual and methodological issues are relevant. These have been well reviewed elsewhere (Valentino, Eberwine & Barchas, 1987; Conn, 1989; Polak & McGee, 1990).

ISHH and neuropsychiatric disease: principles

Uses of ISHH

With regard to the study of disease, all methodologies detecting an mRNA allow its *location* and *relative or absolute abundance* to be compared between healthy and affected brains; the particular value of ISHH is that these parameters can be determined at a finer spatial resolution than with any other technique, thereby providing regional, cellular and even subcellular information about the mRNA (Figures 4.1 and 4.2). This allows the cells expresssing a gene and thus synthesizing the encoded protein to be determined, something which is not always possible immunocytochemically in the brain because of the

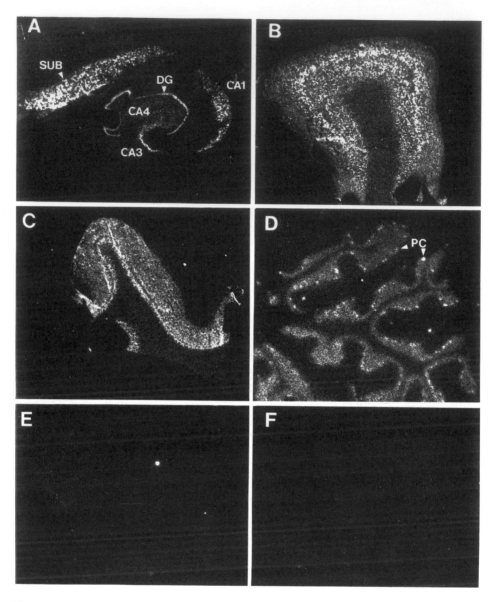

Figure 4.1. Regional distribution of neurofilament (NF-M) mRNA in normal human brain. The patient died from superior vena caval obstruction secondary to bronchial carcinoma; post-mortem interval 7 h. ISHH was carried out as described (see text), using 10^6 cpm of labelled probe, incubated at 28 °C and washed at 54 °C. Sections were exposed to autoradiographic film (Hyperfilm betamax, Amersham) for 28 days. Images are printed directly from film, with increasing whiteness indicating increasing hybridization signal. (A) Hippocampus, showing strong hybridization over the dentate gyrus (DG). Ammon's horn (CA1, CA3, CA4), and subiculum (SUB). (B) Temporal cortex (Brodmann area 21), with accentuation of signal over lamina III. (C) Visual cortex (area 17), with signal concentrated over lamina V/VI. (D) Cerebellum, with strong signal over Purkinje cells (PC). (E) Visual cortex, showing level of background signal seen after hybridization with sense-strand probe. (F) Temporal cortex, showing loss of signal after

transport of proteins within and between cells. For example, ISHH has confirmed that the AD β-amyloid precursor (APP) is produced primarily (though not exclusively) by neurones, which bears upon the likely origin of the APP-derived β/A4 peptide, deposited in the disease.

In general, given that all neuropsychiatric disorders are known or suspected to have a characteristic distribution of pathology that is restricted to certain neuronal populations, this accurate spatial detail is essential since it allows changes in gene expression to be correlated with the pathology at the cellular level. For example, the mRNA content of pyramidal neurones has been shown to be affected by the presence of a neurofibrillary tangle (Griffin *et al.*, 1990), whilst a second messenger G-protein mRNA shows a regionally selective neuronal increase in AD, which parallels the extent of disease involvement in each area (Harrison *et al.*, 1991*a*). Moreover, in a disease such as AD where neuronal loss and gliosis occur, any method not detecting mRNA on a 'per cell' basis, will produce results that reflect, at least in part, the change in number and proportion of constituent cells. ISHH also allows the intracellular distribution of an mRNA to be identified. For example, some mRNAs are present in dendrites as well as in the soma of a neurone, a spatial organization that is gene specific, which may change during development, and, potentially, in the course of a disease. This would have functional implications, given that the production and distribution of the encoded protein are likely to be affected in parallel.

In tandem with its spatial precision, ISHH shares with all hybridization methodologies a high degree of molecular specificity. Thus, it allows the selective detection and quantification of an mRNA giving rise to a single gene product. Such molecular specificity is often unattainable at the protein level. Furthermore, it is increasingly apparent that protein subtypes defined in terms of biochemical properties do not always correspond to distinct gene products. For example, muscarinic cholinergic receptors were previously subdivided according to their ligand binding affinities, whereas it is now possible to classify them in terms of their distinct encoding genes (currently five members, m1–m5). Since ISHH detects the transcripts themselves, the precise localization of cells expressing each receptor gene, and the relative abundance of each mRNA, can be determined without the uncertainty caused by ligands that may not be wholly specific. For example, in AD, muscarinic receptor binding studies have produced somewhat equivocal data but generally find little alteration; in contrast, an ISSH study detecting solely the mRNA encoding the m1 receptor shows a significant increase in AD (Harrison *et al.*, 1991*b* and unpublished observations). Although several explanations for this discrepancy exist, it is possible that the failure to see changes at the protein level is due to differential changes in muscarinic receptor subtypes; ISHH studies detecting m2–m5 receptor mRNAs in AD will help clarify the issue.

---

ribonuclease pretreatment of section. Probe specificity was further confirmed by a Northern blot, which showed a single band of predicted size (3.3 kb).

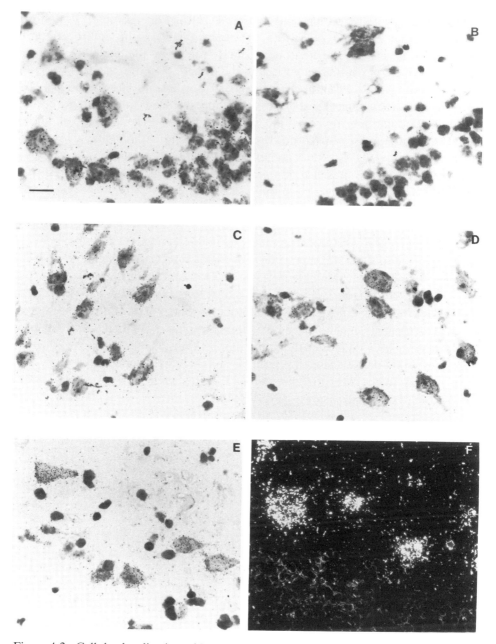

Figure 4.2. Cellular localization of NF-M mRNA in photomicrographs of sections from the case in Figure 4.1. Sections were dipped in Ilford K5 emulsion (see text), exposed for 56 days, developed, and counterstained lightly with toluidine blue. (A) Dentate gyrus/CA4. (B) Dentate gyrus/CA4 from adjacent section after sense-strand hybridization. (C) CA3. (D) CA1. (E) Temporal cortex (area 21), lamina V. (F) Dark field view of Purkinje cells in cerebellum. In (A), (C), (D) and (E), note the concentration of signal over pyramidal neurones. In (F), note that the silver grains are highlighted by the dark field illumination; this is a useful property when considering the measurement of cellular grain density (see text). Scale bar: 25 μm.

The molecular specificity of hybridization extends to allow the differential detection of isoforms, whereby a single gene gives rise to two or more mRNAs by alternative splicing. Again, the encoded proteins may not be distinguishable experimentally, whereas the mRNAs can be, using probes specific for each isoform. Given that splicing patterns for a particular gene are often anatomically specific, developmentally regulated, and affected by disease, this ability of ISHH may prove particularly useful. For example, the microtubule-associated protein *tau* is a major constituent of AD neurofibrillary tangles; it is expressed as at least six mRNAs whose ratio changes through development and, possibly, in the course of the disease. ISHH has already shown the cellular pattern of *tau* mRNA distribution (Kosik *et al.*, 1989) and a localized overall increase in AD hippocampus (Barton *et al.*, 1990); these studies could be extended to look at each individual isoform. Similarly, several members of the non-NMDA (*N*-methyl-D-aspartate) glutamate receptor family are each expressed as one of two isoforms, differing in their intra-hippocampal location and timing of expression (Monyer, Seeburg & Wisden, 1991); not only is this ISHH-derived information of basic neurobiological interest, but may also be of relevance to schizophrenia, in which one of the mRNAs is reduced in a manner suggesting that differential changes in these isoforms might be occurring in the disease (Harrison, McLaughlin & Kerwin, 1991*d*).

Theoretical limitations of ISHH

Detection of an mRNA by ISHH, or by similar methodologies, indicates only that the mRNA was present at the moment of death. Every conclusion beyond this one requires assumptions made with varying degrees of confidence.

It is entirely reasonable to conclude from detection of an mRNA that the gene was being expressed in the tissue, and also to presume that the encoded protein was being synthesized, since an mRNA is, essentially, only present if both transcription and translation are occurring (though there are exceptions to these rules). However, a *change* in amount of an mRNA need not be accompanied by an equivalent change in the rate of synthesis of the encoded protein. Although a relationship of this kind is accepted as a general principle (and is the primary justification for all quantitative assessments of RNA), it is not invariably true. Exceptions in either direction may occur, i.e. parameters of mRNA might change in the absence of an alteration in protein synthesis, and vice versa. For example, it is known that there are active and inactive pools of mRNA within the cell, and regulation of protein synthesis may occur by a change in the relative sizes of this pool without affecting the overall quantity of the mRNA. Alternatively, the rate of protein synthesis per mRNA molecule per unit time might be variable. Such considerations are particularly relevant in the study of neuropsychiatric diseases, since some evidence suggests that the relationship between mRNA and protein may indeed be altered (e.g. Langstrom *et al.*, 1989). Thus, demonstration of a change in the steady state level of an mRNA should be followed by attempts to establish the rate of synthesis and amount of the encoded protein, in order to appreciate the biological significance of the altered mRNA content. Equally, the fact that the amount of an mRNA may be *unchanged* does not imply that expression of that gene is normal, since significant alterations could easily occur in the absence of a change present or detectable at the mRNA level.

Turning to the dynamic nature of gene expression, methods such as ISHH, measuring the abundance of an mRNA, provide no information as to the processes that determine the presence of the mRNA, nor of the mechanisms which might account for a change in amount of the mRNA from one situation to another. Possible explanations for the latter include alterations in rate of transcription or in the rate of mRNA degradation. These aspects of gene expression are technically more complex to investigate, and most are unsuitable for use on post-mortem human brain; however, they should be considered as part of the complete understanding of the role of mRNA in disease. Further discussion of these topics is given by Hargrove & Schmidt (1989) and Wiesner & Zak (1991).

In total, these considerations emphasize that ISHH, like any other single technique, should be used with an awareness of its uses and theoretical limitations, and preferably in conjunction with additional methodologies. There are also practical limitations to the technique, which are discussed below. However, having made these reservations, ISHH remains a valuable tool for providing at least a first step in the understanding of changes in gene expression that may occur in the brain as the result of disease.

Current ISHH data

ISHH in both qualitative and quantitative modes has already been used extensively in the study of AD, and to a much lesser degree in other neuropsychiatric disorders. To date, it is changes in amounts of mRNAs that seem to characterize these diseases, rather than absolute differences in their localization. The theoretical limitations of measurement of mRNA in this way have been referred to above; the practical considerations are discussed in the next section. Quantitative ISHH studies in neuropsychiatry are summarized in Table 4.1 and many are also mentioned in the text to illustrate particular points.

ISHH and neuropsychiatric disease: practice

The possible uses of ISHH in this field have been summarized above. In order for this potential to be fulfilled, a number of practical issues must be addressed relating to the use of human brain tissue.

Table 4.1. *Summary of quantitative changes in mRNAs occurring in neuropsychiatric disorders as identified by ISHH*

mRNA detected[a]	Change in disease[b]	Region[c]	Reference
Alzheimer's disease			
Total APP	Increased	N.basalis	Cohen *et al.*, 1988
	Increased	Subiculum, entorhinal ctx	Higgins *et al.*, 1988
	Unchanged	Visual ctx	Palmert *et al.*, 1988
APP695[d]	Increased	N. basalis, locus coeruleus	Palmert *et al.*, 1988
	Decreased	Hippocampus	Johnson *et al.*, 1990
	Unchanged	N.basalis	Neve *et al.*, 1990
APP563	Increased	N.basalis	Neve *et al.*, 1990
Tau	Increased	Hippocampus	Barton *et al.*, 1990
	Unchanged	Cerebellum	Barton *et al.*, 1990
β-tubulin	Increased	Hippocampus	Geddes *et al.*, 1990
Neurofilament (NF-L)	Decreased[e]	Hippocampus, cerebellum	Somerville *et al.*, 1991
NGF	Increased	N.basalis	Ernfors *et al.*, 1990
receptor	Decreased[f]	N.basalis	Higgins & Mufson, 1989
	Decreased	N.basalis	Neve *et al.*, 1990
Muscarinic m1 receptor	Increased	Temporal ctx	Harrison *et al.*, 1991a
G protein ($G_s\alpha$)	Increased	Hippocampus, temporal ctx	Harrison *et al.*, 1991b
	Unchanged	Visual ctx, cerebellum	Harrison *et al.*, 1991b
Glutamate	Increased	Hippocampus	Harrison *et al.*, 1990
receptor (Glu-R1)	Unchanged	Cerebellum	Harrison *et al.*, 1990
Superoxide	Decreased[e]	Hippocampus	Somerville *et al.*, 1991
dismutase	Unchanged[e]	Cerebellum	Somerville *et al.*, 1991
Pro-opio-melanocortin	Unchanged	Pituitary	Mengod *et al.*, 1991
Poly(A)$^+$	Decreased	Hippocampus, temporal ctx, cerebellum	Harrison *et al.*, 1991c
	Unchanged	Visual ctx	Harrison *et al.*, 1991c
Parkinson's disease			
Tyrosine hydroxylase	Decreased	Substantia nigra	Javoy-Agid *et al.*, 1990
Pro-opio-melanocortin	Unchanged	Pituitary	Mengod *et al.*, 1991
Motor neurone disease			
Neurofilament (NF-L)	Unchanged	Spinal cord	Clark *et al.*, 1990

Table 4.1. *(cont.)*

mRNA detected[a]	Change in disease[b]	Region[c]	Reference
Schizophrenia			
Glutamate receptor (Glu-R1)	Decreased	Hippocampus	Harrison *et al.*, 1991*d*
Pro-opio-melano-cortin	Unchanged	Pituitary	Mengod *et al.*, 1991

Only published quantitative ISHH studies are included. Some use other quantitative methodologies in addition to ISHH.

[a]APP: β-amyloid precursor protein; APP695, APP563: specific APP transcripts; NF-L: neurofilament (light chain); NGF: nerve growth factor; glu-R1: a member of the non-NMDA glutamate receptor gene family.

[b]Compared to normal controls, unless stated.

[c]Either per constituent cell population, or in the region as a whole. The precise method of quantitation varies between studies. ctx, cortex; N. basalis, basal nucleus of Meynert and associated cholinergic forebrain nuclei.

[d]Relative to other APP transcripts, or to total APP mRNA.

[e]Relative to Huntington's chorea cases.

[f]Number of positively labelled cells.

Problems with the use of human brain tissue for RNA research

In comparison with experimental animal brains, there are several additional variables to be taken into account when using post-mortem human tissue to study RNA, whether by ISHH or other methodologies. These are largely to do with the peri-mortem period, and potentially confound the detection and interpretation of changes occurring as a result of the underlying disease.

Post-mortem interval

The post-mortem interval (PMI), in this context, is the time between death and freezing or fixation of the tissue. Since mRNA has a turnover of minutes or hours *in vivo*, it was unclear whether methodologies such as ISHH, relying on preservation of mRNA, could be carried out in human tissue where a PMI of several hours is usually inevitable. In fact, studies have shown that RNA, including intact and biologically active mRNA, is present at essentially un-changed levels even after PMIs of 36–48 h or more, and human brains frozen after a PMI of this magnitude have been used successfully for the whole range of RNA-based methodologies (see Harrison & Pearson, 1990; Harrison *et al.*, 1991*c*). This unexpected stability of RNA after death probably results from rapid inactivation of ribonucleases that normally degrade it. In our ISHH studies, we have found no significant correlations between PMI (range 6 to 48 or 72 h) and the quantity of any specific mRNA (Harrison *et al.*, 1990, 1991*a*, *b*) or of total polyadenylated mRNA (Harrison *et al.*, 1991*c*). Other groups have also found a similar lack of correlation with PMI, and have performed ISHH successfully on tissue after PMIs up to 48h or more (see e.g. Ernfors *et al.*, 1990; Mengod *et al.*, 1990, 1991; Rance & Young, 1991).

These data do not imply that mRNA is impervious to PMI. In most (but not all: see Johnson, Morgan & Finch, 1986) animal studies, a decline – in terms of total RNA, total mRNA, or specific mRNAs – occurs across a PMI range of approximately 4–48 h; the precise temporal pattern and magnitude of decay is unclear and appears to vary depending upon methodology and the RNA parameter being measured (e.g. Barton & Hardy, 1987; Rivkees *et al.*, 1989; Noguchi, Arai & Iizuka, 1991; Somerville *et al.*, 1991). Moreover, in our human ISHH studies, negative correlations between PMI and signal strength are usually observed, but do not reach significance. Certainly, the PMI should be matched between disease and control groups, and separate correlations with PMI determined for each group to exclude the theoretical possibility that there is an interaction of PMI with pre-existing brain disease. It should also be noted that ISHH does not necessarily indicate that the mRNA is intact, only that fragments of similar length to the probe are present; however, there is little or no evidence for partial degradation of mRNA even at prolonged PMIs, with most data indicating that RNA is either intact or wholly degraded.

Agonal state

That the effect of PMI on RNA is generally more apparent in brains from experimental animals than from humans may be due to species differences. Much more likely, it reflects the many other variables present in the latter situation, which mask the contribution of PMI to RNA detection. Of these, the pre-mortem course (agonal state) is probably most important. As with some neurochemical measures, mRNA appears to be susceptible to phenomena such as hypoxia, acidosis and pyrexia, which are variable occurrences before death. For example, the amount of muscarinic receptor mRNA detected by ISHH declines with increasing duration of terminal coma (likely to be accompanied by hypoxia) in a series of dementia cases (Harrison *et al.*, 1991*c*), whilst APP mRNAs are differentially affected by hypoxia (Abe, Tanzi & Kogure, 1991). However, other mRNAs appear to be unaffected by agonal state (e.g. Harrison *et al.*, 1991*a*), indicating that this factor is likely to be restricted to a subpopulation of mRNAs. Thus, the agonal state should be documented and preferably matched at least approximately between groups, with its influence being determined for each transcript to be investigated. This is especially relevant for the study of diseases such as Alzheimer's disease, whose sufferers tend to die agonally, whereas a series of normal controls may include a higher proportion of rapid deaths.

In summary, both PMI and agonal state may affect subsequent detection of RNA and need to be considered carefully when carrying out ISHH and related techniques. However, their effects in no way preclude the use of post-mortem tissue for ISHH or other RNA research.

Other factors

Two further factors affecting RNA are relevant. Firstly, the quantity and distribution of specific mRNAs are often affected by both short-term and long-term medication (e.g. psychotropics, steroids), and the patient's drug history should therefore also be taken into account. Secondly, all post-mortem studies show that there is a significant variability in RNA content and integrity between human brains, which exceeds that seen with animal tissue, and which remains unexplained. For example, some brains contain very little intact RNA, even after a short PMI and apparently rapid death, and average human brain RNA yields are always lower than from rat brain. It is assumed, although unproven, that a combination of individual pre-mortem factors accounts for much of the variability. Whatever the reason, it makes methodologies such as ISHH unsuitable for detecting minor disease-related changes in mRNAs, since the brain-to-brain variability will preclude their detection unless unrealistically large sample sizes are used. Identification of the factors accounting for the variance in mRNA content between brains would be a major advance in this field; in the meantime, a number of strategies have been employed to at least partially overcome the problem (see below).

Methodological issues

The recognition of, and allowance for, the effects of agonal state and PMI are the main additional factors to consider when planning ISHH for use with human as opposed to animal brain tissue. In consequence, it is the availability of a suitably documented, matched and processed series of brains which, to a large extent, sets the upper limit upon the quality and strength of the resulting data. The value of close co-operation between psychiatrist or neurologist, pathologist and the research team is apparent; in comparison, the ISHH methodology itself can be relatively straightforward.

For those interested in neuropathological research, ISHH will be used as an investigative tool, and what is required is a successful and simple methodology that allows not only the localization of specific mRNAs but also their relative quantities to be determined and compared with controls for the disease in question. The ISHH methodology we have applied to human brain for these purposes derives from this philosophy. It uses ^{35}S-labelled synthetic oligonucleotide probes to detect specific mRNAs in frozen tissue sections and is suitable for both human and experimental animal work. The protocol has been documented elsewhere (Harrison & Pearson, 1990; Najlerahim *et al.*, 1990),

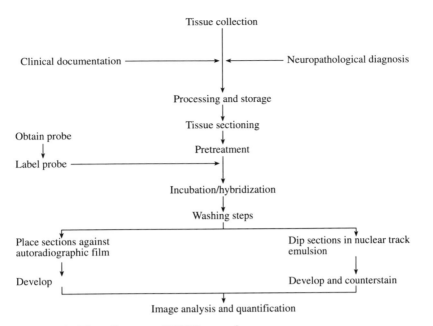

Figure 4.3. Flow diagram of ISHH procedures.

and the procedural sequence is illustrated in Figure 4.3. The following discussion mentions specific areas that either have received little attention in the literature or that can cause difficulty; the options for each step are also outlined, and have been discussed in more detail by Harrison & Pearson (1990).

Tissue processing and preparation

Most ISHH work in this field has used post-fixed frozen tissue, although the whole range of embedding and fixation methods have been used successfully. What is important is that a suitable processing protocol is established, and is identical for each brain, since, for example, even minor variations in fixation parameters affect hybridization signal (Valentino *et al.*, 1987, and our unpublished observations). Successful ISHH using routine formalin-fixed paraffin-embedded sections has been demonstrated (e.g. Somerville *et al.*, 1991), but generally the sensitivity is lower than with frozen tissue, and additional processing steps prior to ISHH are required.

There is little evidence that mRNA decays even over a prolonged period (i.e. several years) if tissue is stored at −70 °C or in paraffin blocks, although it is sensible to check for an effect of this variable. RNA does not appear to be so stable in tissue sections: it is lost within weeks from frozen sections if they are not post-fixed; even after fixation, signal from such sections shows a significant decline after storage of more than two years or so (unpublished observations). Thus, the bulk of tissue should be stored as blocks rather than as sections.

Choice of probes

Oligonucleotides are short DNA probes that have advantages over other probe types in terms of ease and cost of acquisition and of use. They are suitable for most experimental purposes, although unlike other probe types they require that the sequence of the target transcript is known in order to synthesize a probe with the correct sequence; given their short length (around 30–45 bases), exact matching is essential. A number of experimental controls are also required (see below).

Complementary DNA (cDNA) and cRNA ('riboprobes') probes require molecular biological expertise for their synthesis, and are technically more difficult to use, especially the latter. However, they can be labelled to a higher specific activity, giving a stronger ISHH signal, and their length makes the resulting hybrids inherently more specific.

Choice of label

Both radioactive and non-radioactive labelling of probes has been used for ISHH. The commonest radioactive label is ^{35}SdATP, since ^{35}S allows accurate localization of signal with a reasonably short autoradiographic exposure. Other labels that can be used are ^{3}H, ^{32}P and ^{125}I. As a rule, non-radioactive methods have been less sensitive than radioactive ISHH, and the resulting signal is more difficult to quantitate or standardize, limiting their use in neuropathological research. However, recent data attest to their improvements, and they are likely to become increasingly popular, given the shorter exposure times and greater safety than radioactive methods (e.g. Kiyama, Emson & Tohyama, 1990; Larsson & Hougaard, 1990; Augood et al., 1991).

Autoradiographic detection of signal

Figures 4.1 and 4.2 demonstrate the results of ISHH as detected on autoradiographic film and with liquid emulsion respectively. Using film allows the *regional* distribution of the mRNA to be determined and compared, for example, between hippocampal CA fields or between cortical laminae. This level of resolution is slightly more focussed than a regional Northern blot, and can provide valuable information (e.g. Harrison et al., 1991b, c). It also allows the success of an ISHH experiment to be established more easily than with liquid autoradiography, as well as indicating the exposure time necessary for the latter (about three times as long as that needed for optimal film exposure).

Liquid emulsion autoradiography ('dipping') is technically difficult, irreversible, and more time-consuming than film autoradiography. However, it is the only means for *cellular* localization and quantitation of an mRNA that has been detected using radioactive methods, and is therefore essential if this particular advantage of ISHH is to be utilized. Its technical problems are especially relevant if quantitation is to be carried out, since the formation of silver grains is affected by factors such as emulsion thickness and level of background signal, both of which are subject to experimental variation and artefact. Suitable emulsions, such as Ilford K5 or Amersham LM1, include detailed instructions for their use. The emulsions are extremely light-sensitive, and rigorous attention must be paid to darkroom conditions. All sections from a given experiment should be dipped in an identical fashion during a single session, with each batch including blank slides and unhybridized sections to determine background grain density and to exclude chemographic artefacts. Further discussion of autoradiographic principles and practice is given by Rogers (1979).

Experimental controls for oligonucleotide ISHH

A number of controls are needed to ensure that the signal is due entirely to specific hybridization to the desired target mRNA.

Search of gene databases

Although not strictly a control, before obtaining an oligonucleotide it is sensible to check that the proposed sequence, or one similar to it, is not contained in any other known transcript that might be expressed in the brain. This is achieved by running the sequence against a gene database, such as that held by the European Molecular Biology Organization, which can be accessed through terminals in many biochemistry departments. A negative result by no means excludes the presence of such additional transcripts (given that many human genes remain unsequenced), but at least the likelihood can be reduced.

Northern blotting

A Northern blot contains total RNA extracted from a tissue that has been separated electrophoretically by size on a gel, and transferred to a filter. If the filter is incubated with a labelled probe under suitable conditions, hybridization will occur to the target RNA species, if it is present, and which is detected as a black band after placing the hybridized filter against autoradiographic film. The molecular size of the target mRNA can be estimated relative to the 28 S and 18 S rRNA bands, or by loading one lane of the gel with RNA of known sizes.

Northern blotting (or Northern analysis) is a necessary control for oligonucleotide ISHH, since it is possible (despite the use of a gene database) that the nucleotide sequence complementary to the oligonucleotide is, unknowingly, contained in another brain mRNA. This will result in an ISHH picture that reflects the distribution of all such transcripts. Thus, the intended oligonucleotide probe is first hybridized to a Northern blot containing RNA from human brain, preferably from the region(s) to be studied by ISHH. If a single band is seen, corresponding to the known size of the target mRNA, it can be assumed that the probe is detecting only the desired mRNA *in situ*. If two or more bands are observed, these may correspond to alternative splice products of the target mRNA, but if this cannot be confirmed, another oligonucleotide should be chosen and the process repeated. Similarly, if a band is seen that is close in size to that of the rRNA bands, hybridization may be occurring to rRNA rather than to mRNA. This possibility can be excluded by loading the gel prior to blotting with polyadenylated (poly(A)$^+$) mRNA rather than total RNA, thus removing the rRNA: if, after hybridization, the band is still present, it can be concluded that the probe is detecting mRNA and not rRNA.

Sense-strand hybridization

Regardless of probe type, it is valuable to have a control that indicates the degree of non-specific binding *in situ*. This is usually obtained by the concurrent use on adjacent sections of a sense-strand probe, i.e., one whose sequence is identical, not complementary, to the target mRNA, and which therefore cannot hybridize to it. (The complementary probe that does detect the target mRNA is called the antisense probe; Figure 4.4.) Any signal arising from the sense strand is assumed to be non-specific, and can be subtracted from that seen with the antisense probe if quantitation is to be performed. Occasionally, sense-strand hybridization produces a strong signal, probably due to hybridization to rRNA, and requires that a new pair of probes is obtained.

A similar form of control to a sense strand is given by reverse antisense (where the sequence is identical with the antisense probe but in the opposite orientation, again precluding hybridization; Figure 4.4), or by the use of 'nonsense' probes (which are not complementary to any known transcript).

Ribonuclease pretreatment

RNAase pretreatment (Najlerahim *et al.*, 1990) prior to ISHH is intended to remove RNA from the section and thus abolish subsequent signal, so demonstrating that the latter is due to detection of RNA (Figure 4.1F). This is an essential control if a sense or reverse antisense strand is not used. In practice, a small (but variable) amount of signal often remains after ribonuclease, presumably due to incomplete digestion of the mRNA; however, the signal intensity should be greatly reduced.

Sense strand	5'–ACU GGC CCC AUU–3'
Antisense strand	3'–TGA CCG GGG TAA–5'
Reverse antisense	5'–TGA CCG CCC TAA–3'

Figure 4.4. Nomenclature of probe orientations. Note that the antisense strand is shown in the 3'–5' direction for convenience. The sense strand is, by definition, identical to the target mRNA sequence, although the latter contains uridine instead of thymidine residues, since it is RNA not DNA.

'Cold displacement'

This refers to the loss of signal seen due to competition if incubation is carried out in the presence of an excess ($\times 50$) of unlabelled antisense probe. This demonstrates that signal arises from specific binding (i.e. hybridization), and is analogous to the form of control used in ligand-binding studies.

Varying the incubation temperature

This also serves as a form of control, since hybrid stability is temperature dependent, as described by the formula:

$$T_m = 16.6 \log[M] + 0.41[P_{GC}] + 81.5 - [P_m] - 675/L - 0.65[P_f]$$

where: T_m is the melt temperature, at which 50% of hybrids are predicted to dissociate, $[M]$ is the molar concentration of sodium in the solution, to a maximum of 0.5 M, $[P_{GC}]$ is the percentage of bases in the probe that are guanine or cytosine, $[P_m]$ is the percentage of mismatches between probe and target sequence, L is the probe length in bases, and $[P_f]$ is the percentage formamide in the solution.

Incubation and washing steps are generally carried out at 15 °C below T_m. If the temperature is raised towards and beyond T_m, signal strength should decline predictably, further indicating that signal derives from specific hybridization. (This formula also demonstrates that, for oligonucleotides, even a small mismatch from 100% homology will weaken hybridization; for a 30mer, each non-complementary base reduces the T_m by about 3 °C.)

Summary

By virtue of their short length, oligonucleotide probes need rigorous experimental controls to ensure the specificity of the ISHH picture. As a minimum, each probe should be subject to Northern analysis, and every ISHH experiment should be accompanied by sense-strand hybridization carried out under identical conditions. If there is any doubt about the results, additional controls such as ribonuclease pretreatment and cold displacement should be used. It may also be valuable to repeat the experiment using another oligonucleotide directed against a separate part of the same mRNA, in order to demonstrate that an identical distribution of signal is seen; this greatly reduces any likelihood that either probe is inadvertently detecting an additional transcript. For cDNA and cRNA probes, there is less need for multiple controls, especially Northern analysis, and sense-strand hybridization alone is often sufficient.

Quantification of ISHH

The rationale for, and limitations of measuring RNA levels have been discussed above. Notwithstanding the theoretical considerations, this section discusses the practical issues that at least can make the process feasible and reliable for ISHH.

With regard to the study of neuropsychiatric disease, quantitative ISHH, at its simplest, compares signal strength between cases and controls. If there is a difference, it is taken to indicate that the amount of the mRNA is similarly altered, since signal strength is in some way proportional to the amount of mRNA present (assuming uniform experimental conditions and an excess of probe). This most basic form of relative quantification can be applied either to autoradiographic film (e.g. to compare signal strength measured densitometrically over the cortical grey matter in AD: Harrison *et al.*, 1991a), or to 'per cell' quantification, when the densitometric value is a measure of the number of silver grains over the cell (e.g. Harrison *et al.*, 1991a, c).

For quantification of either autoradiographic film or dipped sections, the procedure is generally carried out using a computerized image analysis system, of which several are now available. Manual cellular grain counts can also be performed. All image analysis systems in this context rely on the principle that they register the transmission of light through a piece of film or a slide, and that the resulting numerical value reflects the 'grey density' of the object, which is in turn determined by the ISHH signal. Such procedures clearly require that the system is suitably set up, with constant illumination and standard conditions.

It is possible to get beyond simple densitometric measurements and to calibrate the initial grey-density scale, for instance in terms of concentration of radioactivity or of target mRNA. The simplest calibration is to use plastic autoradiographic standards of known radioactivity, which are exposed against film along with the sections; this allows densitometric results to be converted to units of radioactivity per unit mass. An example of this procedure is illustrated in Figure 4.5. The same principle can be accomplished by embedding known concentrations of the radioactive ligand in a medium such as brain paste, allowing sections to be cut which are then exposed along with the experimental sections (e.g. Miller, Urban & Dorsa, 1989). Such manoeuvres allow the sizes of changes of grey density registered by the image analyser to be expressed in terms of, say, a doubling of radioactivity. This, however, still does not imply a doubling of mRNA concentration in the tissue. An approximation to the latter can be obtained by embedding a known concentration of unlabelled sense-strand in brain paste and hybridizing to sections cut from this. If a range of sense-strand concentrations are used, densitometric values can be converted to amount of mRNA (strictly, sense-strand equivalents) per unit mass of tissue or protein (e.g. Mengod *et al.*, 1991).

Each of these refinements provides additional information about the extent of the change detected by ISHH, and the decision about which to use depends upon whether the increased information justifies the additional input required. In some situations, it may be sufficient merely to show that hybridization signal is increased in a disease, regardless of magnitude, whereas in other circumstances, the size of the change may be important. However, even if calibrated quantification along these lines is achieved, several problems remain. Firstly,

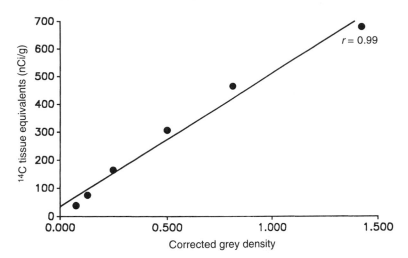

Figure 4.5. A series of [^{14}C] standards ([^{35}S] standards are not available due to its short half-life) of known radioactivity were exposed to autoradiographic film together with experimental ISHH sections. The image analysis system used (Image Manager PC, Sight Systems, Newbury, UK) was programmed to measure the grey density of each standard using an arbitrary scale from 0 (black, maximum signal) to 255 (white, no signal). It was established that a logarithmic transformation of the original grey-density values (specifically, $\log_{10}$[255/grey density]), called 'corrected grey density', produced a linear scale over the range measured, whereby a doubling of radioactivity corresponded to an approximate doubling of corrected grey density. (This exact relationship may not hold under other conditions or for other image-analysis systems that vary in their response properties, and for which a separate transformation may be required.)

none of these methods allows grain densities per neurone to be converted to biologically meaningful units, although it may be assumed that a doubling of grain count indicates at least approximately a doubling of the cellular content of that mRNA, especially if the mean cell size (usually approximated by the area measured by the image analysis system) is shown not to differ between the two situations (e.g. Somerville *et al*., 1991). Secondly, no suitable method currently allows ISHH signal to be understood in terms of copy numbers of mRNA molecules per region or per cell, which is the ultimate goal (see Thompson & Gillespie, 1990).

More generally, the corroboration of ISHH data with other methodologies strengthens the quantitative conclusions that can be drawn, particularly as to the magnitude of the change. For example, Neve, Rogers & Higgins (1990) used ISHH in conjunction with two other techniques to show an increase in specific APP mRNA isoform in Alzheimer's disease. Other techniques that are suitable for quantification of mRNA are solution hybridization and RT-PCR (see Becker-André & Hahlbrock, 1989; Wiesner & Zak, 1991). It should be noted, however, that ISHH may detect genuine alterations that cannot be seen with other techniques, which all rely on extraction of RNA. This is particularly true if a change is restricted to a subpopulation of neurones within an area. For instance, if an mRNA is increased 50% in pyramidal neurones of CA3 field, but not in any other cell type or hippocampal region, then analysis based upon homogenization of the hippocampus is unlikely to detect this change.

The quantification of ISHH is a complex subject, with a number of other aspects and approaches not mentioned here. For more detailed discussion of the conceptual and methodological issues, see Rogers, Schwaber & Lewis (1987); Conn (1989); McCabe, Desharnais & Pfaff (1989); Nunez *et al*. (1989); Uhl (1989) and Young (1989), as well as Chapter 11.

Quantification relative to overall mRNA content

Gene expression as a whole, whether measured in terms of a parameter of total RNA content or otherwise, varies in response to diverse biological and pathological stimuli. Thus, it is valuable to relate a change in a single mRNA to an indicator of overall gene expression in order to ascertain the molecular specificity of the change. Such markers may be provided by expressing data as a percentage of an RNA species that does not appear to vary between situations; β-actin mRNA or rRNA are often used. Alternatively, total poly(A)$^+$ mRNA may be estimated using a probe detecting the poly(A) tails common to the majority of individual mRNAs. The amount of a given mRNA can then be normalized to the quantity of poly(A)$^+$ mRNA detected by ISHH in the same region or cell population of each brain (Griffin, 1987). This method has been applied to show increases in specific mRNAs in AD (Barton *et al*., 1990; Harrison *et al*., 1991*a, b*) against a background of reduced poly(A)$^+$ mRNA content (Harrison *et al*., 1991*c*). Finally, a different type of internal standard is to measure an mRNA in two cell populations within the same region, and express them as a ratio; this method partially overcomes the problems of varying RNA content, caused both by genuine and experimental factors, and has been used to show a differential change in APP mRNA between hippocampal subfields in AD (Higgins *et al*., 1988).

Extensions of ISHH

In some circumstances it may be valuable to establish whether two mRNAs are expressed in the same cell and the extent to which their precise distribution overlaps. This can be achieved by double-labelling ISHH, whereby one transcript is detected autoradiographically, and the other by a non-radioactive method (e.g. Kiyama *et al*., 1990; Young & Hsu, 1990). Similarly, an mRNA can be co-localized with a protein by sequential ISHH and immunocytochemistry (in either order), providing additional information about co-regulation of gene expression. One relevant example is that of Schalling *et al*. (1990); the detection of neurofibrillary tangles on AD sections used for ISHH has already been mentioned (Kosik *et al*., 1989; Griffin *et al*., 1990). However, combined techniques are technically difficult and usually less sensitive than either method used alone; it is often sufficient to carry out the procedures separately on serial sections, since this still allows study of their co-localization within the same cell population, albeit not the same cell. (Even the latter may be possible, if an X, Y coordinate stage is used to identify the same neurone on the adjacent section).

Finally, two additional methods exist that have the potential to improve the sensitivity of ISHH. One is the use of a post-hybridization signal amplification step (Hoyland & Freemont, 1991), the other is *in situ* transcription (Tecott, Barchas & Eberwine, 1988). Both may have useful applications in the study of mRNA in human brain.

Summary

The ability of ISHH to identify alterations in the cellular localization and relative quantity of specific mRNAs occurring in the course of neuropsychiatric disease provides a new tool for the study of their molecular pathogenesis, especially since it can be successfully performed on post-mortem human brain tissue. However, careful attention must be paid to both pre- and post-mortem confounding factors that may affect mRNA. The particular value of ISHH in this field is its anatomical resolution, allowing correlations to be made at the level of individual neurones between changes in gene expression and the distribution of neuropathological features of a disorder – or, indeed, indicate potential functional impairments of neurones in the absence of observable neuropathology. As with other RNA-directed methodologies, its molecular specificity and ability to be quantified are also major advantages, permitting quantitative estimates of the expression of individual transcripts to be made, although both theoretical and practical constraints with this procedure must be borne in mind. With adequate attention to its principles and practice, and in conjunction with related techniques, ISHH will remain a valuable tool for research into the molecular basis of neurological and psychiatric disorders.

Acknowledgements

Our experimental work is supported by the Wellcome Trust. P. J. H. was a Medical Research Council Training Fellow.

References

Abe, K., Tanzi, R. E. & Kogure, K. (1991). Selective induction of Kunitz-type protease inhibitor domain-encoding amyloid precursor protein mRNA after persistent focal ischemia in rat cerebral cortex. *Neuroscience Letters*, **125**, 172–4.

Augood, S. J., Kiyama, H., Faull, R. L. M. & Emson, P. C. (1991). Dopaminergic D1 and D2 receptor antagonists decrease prosomatostatic mRNA expression in rat striatum. *Neuroscience*, **44**, 35–44.

Barton, A. J. L. & Hardy, J. A. (1987). Stability of brain RNA post mortem: effect of Alzheimer's disease. *Biochemical Society Transactions*, **15**, 558–9.

Barton, A. J. L., Harrison, P. J., Najlerahim, A. *et al*. (1990). Increased tau messenger RNA in Alzheimer's disease hippocampus. *American Journal of Pathology*, **137**, 497–502.

Becker-André, M. & Hahlbrock, K. (1989). Absolute mRNA quantification using the polymerase chain reaction (PCR). A novel approach by a PCR aided transcript titration assay (PATTY). *Nucleic Acids Research*, **17**, 9437–46.

Clark, A. W., Tran, P. M., Parhad, I. M. *et al*. (1990). Neuronal gene expression in amyotrophic lateral sclerosis. *Molecular Brain Research*, **7**, 75–83.

Cohen, M. L., Golde, T. E., Usiak, M. E. *et al*. (1988). In situ hybridization of nucleus basalis neurons shows increased β-amyloid mRNA in Alzheimer's disease. *Proceedings of the National Academy of Sciences, USA*, **85**, 1227–31.

Conn, P. M. (ed.) (1989). *Gene probes. Methods in neuroscience* (Vol. 1). Academic Press, San Diego.

Crapper McLachlan, D. R. & Lewis, P. N. (1985). Alzheimer's disease: errors in gene expression. *Canadian Journal of Neurological Sciences*, **12**, 1–5.

Ernfors, P., Lindefors, N., Chan-Palay, V. & Persson, H. (1990). Cholinergic neurons of the nucleus basalis express elevated levels of nerve growth factor mRNA in senile dementia of the Alzheimer type. *Dementia*, **1**, 138–45.

Geddes, J. W., Wong, J., Choi, B. H. *et al*. (1990). Increased expression of the embryonic form of a developmentally regulated mRNA in Alzheimer's disease. *Neuroscience Letters*, **109**, 54–61.

Griffin, W. S. T. (1987). Methods for hybridization and quantitation of mRNA in individual brain cells. In *In situ hybridization histochemistry: applications to neurobiology* (ed. K. L. Valentino, J. H. Eberwine & J. D. Barchas), pp. 97–110. Oxford University Press, New York.

Griffin, W. S. T., Ling, C., White, C. L., III & Morrison-Bogorad, M. (1990). Polyadenylated messenger RNA in paired helical filament-immunoreactive neurons in Alzheimer's disease. *Alzheimer's Disease and Associated Disorders*, **4**, 69–78.

Hargrove, J. L. & Schmidt, F. H. (1989). The role of mRNA and protein stability in gene expression. *FASEB Journal*, **3**, 2360–70.

Harrison, P. J. (1993). Alzheimer's disease and chromosome 14: different gene, same process? *British Journal of Psychiatry*, **163**, 2–5.

Harrison, P. J. & Pearson, R. C. A. (1990). In situ hybridization histochemistry and the study of gene expression in the human brain. *Progress in Neurobiology*, **34**, 271–312.

Harrison, P. J., Barton, A. J., Najlerahim, A. & Pearson, R. C. A. (1990). Distribution of a kainate/AMPA receptor mRNA in normal and Alzheimer brain. *NeuroReport*, **1**, 149–52.

Harrison, P. J., Barton, A. J. L., McDonald, B. & Pearson, R. C. A. (1991*a*) Alzheimer's disease: specific increases in a G protein subunit (Gsα) mRNA in hippocampal and cortical neurons. *Molecular Brain Research*, **10**, 71–81.

Harrison, P. J., Barton, A. J., Najlerahim, A. *et al*. (1991*b*). Increased muscarinic receptor messenger RNA in Alzheimer's disease temporal cortex demonstrated by in situ hybridization histochemistry. *Molecular Brain Research*, **9**, 15–21.

Harrison, P. J., Barton, A. J. L., Najlerahim, A. *et al*. (1991*c*) Regional and neuronal reductions of polyadenylated messenger RNA in Alzheimer's disease. *Psychological Medicine*, **21**, 855–66.

Harrison, P. J., McLaughlin, D. & Kerwin, R. W. (1991*d*) Decreased hippocampal expression of a glutamate receptor gene in schizophrenia. *Lancet*, **337**, 450–2.

Harrison, P. J., Procter, A. W., Barton, A. J. L. *et al*. (1991*e*) Terminal coma affects messenger RNA detection in post mortem human temporal cortex. *Molecular Brain Research*, **9**, 161–4.

Higgins, G. A., Lewis, D. A., Bahmanyar, S. *et al.* (1988). Differential regulation of amyloid beta-protein mRNA expression within hippocampal subpopulations in Alzheimer's disease. *Proceedings of the National Academy of Sciences, USA*, **85**, 1297–301.

Higgins, G. A. & Mufson, E. J. (1989) NGF receptor gene expression is decreased in the nucleus basalis in Alzheimer's disease. *Experimental Neurology*, **106**, 222–36.

Hoyland, J. A. & Freemont, A. J. (1991). Investigation of a quantitative post-hybridization signal amplification system for mRNA-oligodeoxyribonucleotide in situ hybridization. *Journal of Pathology*, **164**, 51–8.

Javoy-Agid, F., Hirsch, E. C., Dumas, S. *et al.* (1990). Decreased tryosine hydroxylase messenger RNA in the surviving dopamine neurons of the substantia nigra in Parkinson's disease: an *in situ* hybridization study. *Neuroscience*, **38**, 245–53.

Johnson, S. A., McNeill, T., Cordell, B. & Finch, C. E. (1990). Relation of neuronal APP-751/APP-695 mRNA ratio and neuritic plaque density in Alzheimer's disease. *Science*, **248**, 954–857.

Johnson, S. A., Morgan, D. G. & Finch, C. E. (1986). Extensive post mortem stability of mRNA from rat and human brain. *Journal of Neuroscience Research*, **16**, 267–80.

Kiyama, H., Emson, P. C. & Tohyama, M. (1990) Recent progress in the use of the technique of non-radioactive in situ hybridization histochemistry: new tools for molecular neurobiology. *Neuroscience Research*, **9**, 1–21.

Kosik, K. A., Crandall, J. E., Mufson, E. J. & Neve, R. L. (1989) Tau in situ hybridization in normal and Alzheimer brain: predominant localization in the neuronal somatodendritic compartment. *Annals of Neurology*, **26**, 352–361.

Langstrom, N. S., Anderson, J. P., Lindroos, H. G. *et al.* (1989). Alzheimer's disease-associated reduction of polysomal mRNA translation. *Molecular Brain Research*, **5**, 259–69.

Larsson, L.-I. & Hougaard, D. M. (1990). Optimization of non-radioactive in situ hybridization: image analysis of varying pretreatment, hybridization and probe-labelling conditions. *Histochemistry*, **93**, 347–354.

McCabe, J. T., Desharnais, R. & Pfaff, D. W. (1989). Graphical and statistical approaches to data analysis for *in situ* hybridization. *Methods in Enzymology*, **168**, 822–48.

Mengod, G., Charli, J.-L. & Palacios, J. M. (1990). The use of *in situ* hybridization histochemistry for the study of neuropeptide gene expression in the human brain. *Cellular and Molecular Neurobiology*, **10**, 113–26.

Mengod, G., Vivanco, M. M., Christnacher, A. *et al.* (1991). Study of pro-opiomelanocortin mRNA expression in human postmortem pituitaries. *Molecular Brain Research*, **10**, 129–37.

Miller, M., Urban, J. & Dorsa, D. (1989). Quantification of mRNA in discrete cell groups of brain by *in situ* hybridization histochemistry. In *Gene probes. Methods in neuroscience* (Vol. 1) (ed. P. M. Conn), pp. 164–81, Academic Press, San Diego.

Monyer, H., Seeburg, P. H. & Wisden, W. (1991). Glutamate-operated channels: developmentally early and mature forms arise by alternative splicing. *Neuron*, **6**, 799–810.

Najlerahim, A., Harrison, P. J., Barton, A. J. L. *et al.* (1990). Distribution of messenger RNAs encoding the enzymes glutaminase, aspartate aminotransferase and glutamic acid decarboxylase in rat brain. *Molecular Brain Research*, **7**, 317–33.

Neve, R. L., Rogers, J. & Higgins, G. A. (1990) The Alzheimer amyloid precursor-related transcript lacking the β/A4 sequence is specifically increased in

Alzheimer's disease brain. *Neuron*, **5**, 329–38.

Noguchi, I., Arai, H. & Iizuka, R. (1991). A study on postmortem stability of vasopressin messenger RNA in rat brain compared with those in total RNA and ribosomal RNA. *Journal of Neural Transmission* (General Section), **83**, 171–8.

Nunez, D. J., Davenport, A. P., Emson, P. C. & Brown, M. J. (1989). A quantitative in situ hybridization method using computerised image analysis. *Biochemical Journal*, **263**, 121–7.

Palmert, M. R., Golde, T. E., Cohen, M. L. *et al*. (1988). Amyloid protein precursor messenger RNAs: differential expression in Alzheimer's disease. *Science*, **241**, 1080–4.

Polak, J. M. & McGee, J. O'D (eds.) (1990) *In situ hybridization: principles and practice.*. Oxford University Press, Oxford.

Rance, N. E. & Young, W. S., III (1991). Hypertrophy and increased gene expression of neurons containing neurokinin-B and substance-P messenger ribonucleic acids in the hypothalami of postmenopausal women. *Endocrinology*, **128**, 2239–47.

Rivkees, S. A., Chaar, M. R., Hanley, D. *et al*. (1989). Localization and regulation of vasopressin mRNA in human neurons. *Synapse*, **3**, 246–54.

Rogers, A. W. (1979). *Techniques of Autoradiography*, 3rd edn. Elsevier, Amsterdam.

Rogers, W. T., Schwaber, J. S. & Lewis, M. E. (1987). Quantitation of cellular resolution in situ hybridization histochemistry in brain by image analysis. *Neuroscience Letters*, **82**, 315–20.

Schalling, M., Friberg, K., Seroogy, K. *et al*. (1990). Analysis of expression of cholecystokinin in dopamine cells in the ventral mesencephalon of several species and in humans with schizophrenia. *Proceedings of the National Academy of Sciences, USA*, **87**, 8427–31.

Somerville, M. J., Percy, M. E., Bergeron, C. *et al*. (1991). Localisation and quantitation of 68kDa neurofilament and superoxide dismutase-1 mRNA in Alzheimer brain. *Molecular Brain Research*, **9**, 1–14.

Tecott, L. H., Barchas, J. D. & Eberwine, J. H. (1988). *In situ* transcription: specific synthesis of complementary DNA in fixed tissue sections. *Science*, **240**, 1661–4.

Thompson, J. D. & Gillespie, D. (1990). Current concepts in quantitative molecular hybridization. *Clinical Biochemistry*, **23**, 261–6.

Uhl, G. R. (1989). *In situ* hybridization: quantitation using radiolabeled hybridization probes. *Methods in Enzymology*, **168**, 741–52.

Valentino, K. L., Eberwine, J. H. & Barchas, J. D. (eds.) (1987). *In situ hybridization histochemistry: applications to neurobiology*. Oxford University Press, New York.

Wiesner, R. J. & Zak, R. (1991). Quantitative approaches for studying gene expression. *American Journal of Physiology*, **260**, L179–L188.

Young, W. S., III (1989). *In situ* hybridization histochemical detection of neuropeptide mRNAs using DNA and RNA probes. *Methods in Enzymology*, **168**, 702–10.

Young, W. S., III & Hsu, A. C. (1990). Observations on the simultaneous use of digoxygenin and radiolabelled oligodeoxyribonucleotide probes for hybridization histochemistry. *Neuropeptides*, **18**, 75–85.

5

Immunocytochemistry: a neuropathological perspective

STEPHEN M. GENTLEMAN
and GARETH W. ROBERTS

Over the past 40 years the application of immunocytochemical techniques at both the light and electron microscopic level has provided an invaluable functional aspect to complement the well-established morphological observations of classical neuroanatomy. Modern immunocytochemical methods which have evolved rapidly since the pioneering work of Coons and his colleagues in the early 1940s (Coons, Creech & Jones, 1941), now provide a reliable means of visualizing specific tissue antigens *in situ*.

Whilst there are a number of comprehensive texts available on the subject of immunocytochemistry (e.g. Sternberger, 1979; Polak & Van Noorden, 1986) the aim of this chapter is to provide an overview of some of the fundamental considerations and potential problems that may arise in using this technique at the light microscopy level on tissue sections from the central nervous system. At the end of the chapter the potential role of immunocytochemistry in the rapidly expanding field of quantitative pathology is also discussed.

Optimum conditions for immunocytochemistry are generally derived as the result of a trial and error process. If a protocol works in a particular laboratory it tends to acquire a mystique which presupposes that all the steps are vitally important and should therefore never be changed. To a certain extent this is true and if something works why change it? However, it may save time and money to start from the most basic procedure and add new blocking or improvement steps sequentially. In this way the effect of individual steps can be assessed and redundant procedures can be eliminated. With this in mind a staining protocol routinely used in our own laboratory for work on post-mortem human tissue is described in the appendix to this chapter and is intended to provide a basic framework for people setting up immunocytochemistry from scratch.

Antibodies

Primary antibodies raised against a wide variety of different antigens are available commercially and provide the quickest and cheapest option for immunostaining. However, when an antigen is particularly novel there may not be any commercial antibodies available. At this stage it is often worth writing to other investigators in the field who have their own antibodies, which they may be willing to share. Failing this, antibodies can be produced in the laboratory. The choice then lies between producing polyclonal or monoclonal antibodies, both of which have their own advantages and disadvantages.

Polyclonal antisera contain a mixture of antibodies, produced by different cells, that react specifically with different epitopes on a given antigen. They are most commonly raised in rabbits, which are easy to maintain, but can also be raised in other species. For details of the production of polyclonals see the paper by De Mey & Moeremans (1986). In order to increase the specificity of polyclonal antibodies, antisera can be purified by removing other serum proteins (by ion exchange chromatography) and separation from cross-reacting antibodies (by immunoadsorbent affinity chromatography).

In 1976, Köhler & Milstein developed a method for producing monoclonal antibodies, which recognize a single epitope. The process is more complicated and time consuming than that used to produce polyclonals (see Ritter, 1986, for details) but the end result is a theoretically infinite supply of a homogeneous antibody with absolute specificity. A disadvantage of monoclonals is that the epitope must be unique to the antigen of interest, otherwise there can be problems with cross-reactivity. Furthermore, monoclonals are generally of lower affinity than polyclonals, which means they need to be used at a higher concentration.

When buying antibodies from commercial sources be aware that, however good the quality control, there may be variation in the performance of antibodies from different batches. For this reason it is best to estimate how much antibody you are going to need to complete a study before starting it and then obtain the requisite amount. There is nothing more annoying than having to go through the optimization of staining conditions for a new antibody when you are approaching the end of an extensive study.

Fixation

Successful immunocytochemistry requires that fresh tissues are treated with chemical fixatives to preserve their structure and to prevent the loss of soluble antigens during a staining procedure that often involves a series of vigorous washing steps. Fixatives prevent autolysis by inactivating lysosomal enzymes and form chemical cross-links within the tissue that help to maintain its morphological integrity. They also inhibit bacterial and fungal growth.

There are a number of problems associated with achieving good tissue fixation, not least of which is that cross-linking of fixative molecules may mask antigenic sites or, worse still, cause changes in the chemical structure of the antigen. The smaller the antigen the greater this potential problem becomes. In the end a compromise must be reached between maintaining the morphology of the tissue and retaining the antigen of interest. An example of this delicate balancing act is seen with glutaraldehyde, which is a very effective fixative but tends to mask peptide antigens. A suitable compromise in this case is to include glutaraldehyde in the fixative but at a low concentration (Sloviter & Nilaver, 1987).

There are a wide variety of fixatives available to choose from and to a large extent the choice must be determined empirically. Ultimately the fixative used will depend on the antigen to be detected and the tissue that it is to be located in. Cryostat sections may be pre- or post-fixed, i.e. before or after cutting. Depending on the antigen, almost any fixative can be used for pre-fixation. A particularly useful fixative for brain tissue, that is very easy to prepare fresh, is a 4% (w/v) solution of paraformaldehyde in phosphate-buffered saline. Post-fixation of tissue sections on slides can be achieved using a 15 min incubation in acetone or ethanol. For paraffin sections fixatives such as formalin, Bouin's (a solution containing picric acid and formalin) and periodate-lysine paraformaldehyde solutions can be used. The latter is particularly effective at preserving carbohydrate and lipid antigens (McLean & Nakane, 1974).

Optimal fixation can be achieved in animals by using an intracardial perfusion technique (Palay *et al.*, 1962) that allows rapid fixation of the brain *in situ*, thereby minimizing the mechanical damage that can arise when removing fresh tissue from the cranium. Results can sometimes be further improved by perfusing at different pHs or temperatures. For example, a two-stage perfusion can be employed that involves using a low pH solution initially, to allow rapid penetration of the fixative, followed by a higher pH solution, which increases cross linkage and hence fixation (Berod, Hartman & Pujol, 1981).

For obvious reasons, intracardial perfusion is not appropriate for the collection of human post-mortem material. Consequently, there will always be a disparity in the quality of immunostaining obtained in animal and human tissue. Human brains are routinely fixed by immersion in a 10% (v/v) solution of formalin for up to four weeks. This is not an ideal situation because large blocks of tissue will not allow adequate and even penetration of the fixative. To overcome this problem the brains can be cut into 1 cm slices, which will improve fixative penetration. However, once again a compromise needs to be reached because slicing the brain before fixation can result in tissue distortion caused by the dehydrating action of the fixative.

In both human and animal tissue, inadequate or uneven fixation can result in a loss of antigenicity and patchy inconsistent staining. Variations in fixation time and conditions are the root cause of many of the problems encountered in immunocytochemistry. Consequently, it is well worth spending some time in optimizing this particular stage of the technique. Fixation of human tissue is never going to be as good as that seen in freshly perfused animals but there are ways of improving the chances of obtaining well-fixed tissue. Post-mortem delay should be kept to a minimum. Delays of anything longer than 48 h result in poor, inconsistent immunostaining. Another potentially important factor is the agonal state of the patient ante-mortem, which has recently been shown to affect the levels of mRNA detectable by *in situ* hybridization in the brain (Harrison *et al.*, 1991). Very little has been done to establish the effect of agonal state on immunostaining, presumably because the staining has never been quantified in such a way that any difference could be revealed. Information about post-mortem delay can usually be supplied by brain banks (see Chapter 1).

Tissue processing

When the appropriate tissue has been collected, the next decision to be made concerns the best way to process it. There are a number of different options available for producing tissue sections. Probably the most widely used method for human surgical or post-mortem tissue is paraffin embedding. This involves dehydrating the tissue, embedding in hot paraffin wax and then cutting on a wax microtome. Perhaps not surprisingly, this relatively harsh treatment of the tissue does result in a certain loss of antigenicity for some antigens. However, the morphology of the sections is generally very good, they can be cut reliably at a thickness down to 1–5 μm and in many cases the only material available for retrospective clinical studies comes from pathology laboratories, where this is the standard procedure.

A second option is to use vibratome sections. These can be cut accurately down to a thickness of about 40 μm and are particularly useful for morphological studies where the three-dimensional distribution of the stained features is important. As the sections are relatively thick, they are more effectively treated free-floating than slide mounted. Although this requires the use of larger volumes of antibodies, it does allow access to the tissue from both cut surfaces as opposed to only one. To allow maximal penetration of the antibodies into the tissue, it is often advisable to prolong the incubation of the sections with the primary antibody. Cutting with a vibratome is carried out on unfrozen tissue with no supporting medium. It is therefore essential that the tissue to be cut is of a suitable consistency to be able to stand alone and provide some resistance to the vibrating microtome blade. Well-fixed brain tissue generally meets this criterion.

Cryostat sections have a distinct advantage over paraffin sections in that the processing is less traumatic on the tissue and therefore antigenicity is generally better. However, this is countered to some extent by the fact that tissue morphology is not well preserved in frozen sections. Following fixation, the tissue needs to be rinsed and stored for a minimum of 24 h in phosphate-buffered saline containing 15% (w/v) sucrose and 0.01% (w/v) sodium azide. The sucrose acts as a cryoprotectant, while the sodium azide restricts fungal growth. The blocks are prepared for sectioning by rapid freezing in melting isopropane or Arcton 12 (ICI, UK). Prior to cutting, the blocks are

placed in the cryostat to allow them to equilibrate to the cutting temperature
($-20\,^{\circ}$C). Sections should be collected on pre-washed, adherent coated slides.
The adherent can be a standard histological solution of chrome-alum gelatin or
a high molecular weight polymer such as poly-L-lysine (Huang *et al.*, 1983).
The adherent used will depend on the antigen and antibody in question,
because different adherents may cause different background problems. In some
cases sections may need pretreatment before incubation with the primary
antibody. A common method of aiding antibody penetration into the tissue is
treatment with a detergent such as Triton X-100 (Hartman, Zide & Adenfriend, 1972). This also diminishes background staining and helps to spread
antibody solutions over the tissue. Conversely, dextran sulphate can be used to
raise the surface tension of antibody solutions and stop large sections, for
example of human brain, from drying out (Gentleman *et al.*, 1989*b*). Better
antibody penetration can also be achieved by dehydrating and rehydrating the
tissue through graded alcohol solutions.

If antigens have become masked by fixation, a limited incubation with a
protease such as trypsin may be a useful means of breaking down some of the
fixative cross-links (Huang, Minassian & More, 1976). Care should be taken
not to destroy the tissue and its antigens completely using this approach.
Pretreatment of sections with formic acid is now a widely used method for
unmasking the antigenic sites of central nervous system amyloid deposits
(Kitamoto *et al.*, 1987).

Choice of technique

Immunocytochemistry allows the *in situ* visualization of tissue antigens through
the use of labelled or unlabelled antibodies. In their original experiments,
Coons *et al.* (1941) employed the fluorescent marker fluorescein isothiocyanate
(FITC), which they conjugated directly to a primary antibody. Since then the
technique has been extensively modified to improve both the sensitivity and the
specificity of the immunostaining. Currently, the most widely used methods are
indirect immunofluorescence (Coons, Leduc & Connolly, 1955), indirect peroxidase anti-peroxidase (PAP) (Sternberger, 1979), avidin–biotin complex
(ABC) (Hsu, Raine & Fanger, 1981) and immunogold silver (IGS) (Holgate *et
al*, 1983).

Indirect immunofluorescence is the simplest of the three techniques. With
this method the primary antibody is unlabelled while a secondary antibody,
raised against the immunoglobulin of the first antisera species, is conjugated
with a suitable fluorescent marker (Figure 5.1A). Commonly used fluorophores
include FITC, which fluoresces a yellow-green, rhodamine, Texas red and,
more recently, 7-amino-4-methylcoumarin-3-acetic acid (AMCA), which produces a bright blue fluorescence.

The PAP technique is slightly more complicated in that three different

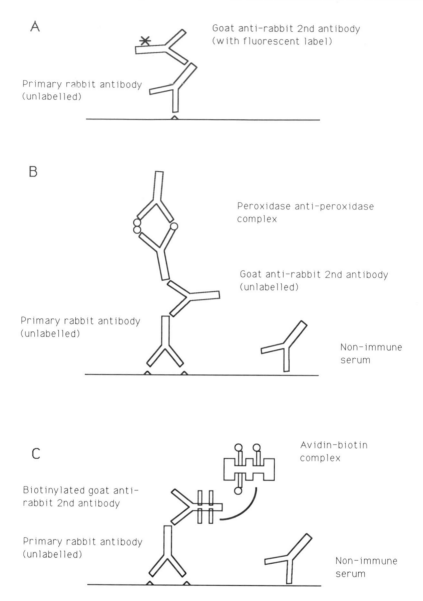

Figure 5.1. Schematic representation of the principles underlying three of the most widely used immunocytochemical techniques. (A) Indirect immunofluorescence using a secondary antibody labelled with a fluorescent marker. (B) Peroxidase anti-peroxidase (PAP) method using an unlabelled secondary antibody and a third-layer antibody/peroxidase complex. (C) Avidin–biotin complex (ABC) method using a biotinylated secondary antibody and a third-layer avidin/biotin/peroxidase complex. In all these methods a preincubation with non-immune serum from the species in which the second-layer antibody was raised will block non-specific binding sites within the tissue. (Adapted from Polak & Van Noorden, 1986.)

antisera are used. The first and second layer antisera are essentially the same as those described for the indirect immunofluorescence method, except that in this case the secondary antiserum is also unlabelled (Figure 5.1B). The third reagent is a peroxidase anti-peroxidase complex composed of antibodies against the enzyme horseradish peroxidase raised in the same species as the primary antiserum and coupled immunologically to the peroxidase enzyme. The enzyme is developed histochemically (Graham & Karnovsky, 1966) to give a dark brown, permanent deposit on the site of the detected antigen. This method is particularly sensitive because the peroxidase is immunologically, rather than chemically, bound to the anti-peroxidase molecule and therefore loses none of its enzymatic activity. The increased amount of label also allows for a higher dilution of the primary antibody, thereby eliminating a large part of the non-specific background staining.

The ABC system relies on the extraordinary high affinity of the 68 kDa glycoprotein avidin, which is found in egg white, for the much smaller vitamin, biotin. As with the PAP method this is a three-layer system but in this case the secondary antisera is labelled with biotin and the third layer contains no antibodies but consists of a preformed complex of avidin and biotin molecules along with a suitable enzyme marker, such as horseradish peroxidase (Figure 5.1C). Initially, when this technique was being developed, there were some problems with avidin in that it binds to non-specific sites within tissues via its carbohydrate moieties. To overcome this problem streptavidin, a bacterial form of the protein that does not bind non-specifically, was introduced. However, modified versions of avidin that give a background staining comparable to streptavidin are now widely available.

IGS is a very sensitive but also relatively expensive technique, which has been adapted from its original use in electron microscopy. Colloidal gold particles are attached to protein A or to immunoglobulins directly (De Mey *et al.*, 1986). Accumulated gold particles can then be seen as a red deposit in the tissue. At this stage the method is no more sensitive than a normal PAP technique, however sensitivity can be greatly increased with a subsequent silver precipitation reaction (Holgate *et al.*, 1983; Springall *et al.*, 1984).

With such a variety of immunostaining techniques available a choice has to be made as to which is the most appropriate for the project in question. Each technique has its own advantages and disadvantages. Immunofluorescence is particularly useful for double immunostaining experiments where different antigens are co-localized in the same cells. It also produces aesthetically pleasing results with regard to photography. However, immunofluorescence is generally less sensitive than the enzymatic methods and it produces staining that fades relatively quickly. Therefore, if long-term image analysis studies are envisaged, a more permanent PAP or ABC immunostain should be used. From our own experience with quantitative pathological studies we have found that, although both methods produce intense immunostaining, the ABC method is appreciably more sensitive than PAP (Figure 5.2).

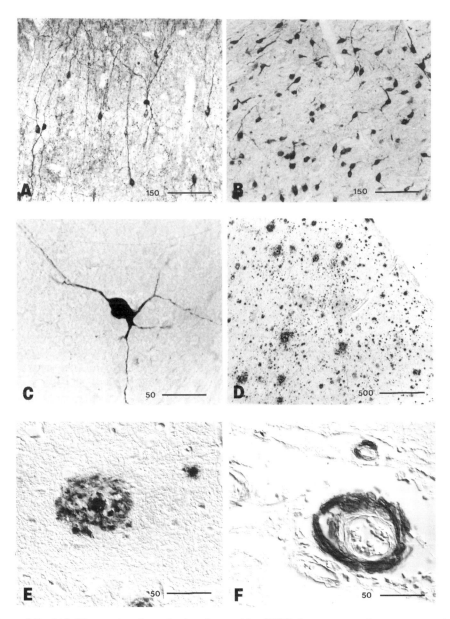

Figure 5.2. (A) Vasoactive intestinal polypeptide (VIP) immunoreactive neurones in the superficial layers of the rat cerebral cortex. (B) Galanin immunoreactive neurones in the human ventral hypothalamus. Comparison of these two photos highlights the difference in morphological definition between perfusion fixed rat tissue and immersion-fixed post-mortem human tissue. (C) A single multipolar neurone from rat cerebral cortex immunostained with a polyclonal antibody to the C-flanking peptide of neuropeptide Y (CPON) showing the fine dendritic staining achieved with the ABC technique described in the appendix. (D), (E) Senile plaques and (F) vascular deposits in the brain from an Alzheimer's disease patient, stained with a monoclonal antibody to the β-amyloid protein. Note the high contrast of the staining, which allows accurate quantification of these characteristic lesions. Scale bars in μm.

Alternative immunoenzyme detection systems

Although horseradish peroxidase was the first enzyme to be introduced for use in immunolabelling (Nakane & Pierce, 1966), there are other enzyme labels available that use different chromogenic reactions to reveal the location of the antigen. With the peroxidase reaction the enzyme donates electrons to hydrogen peroxide. The oxidized enzyme is then restored to its reduced form by the diaminobenzidine (DAB), which acts as an electron donor. The oxidized DAB then rapidly polymerizes to produce a highly insoluble and amorphous brown deposit, which is visible under the light microscope (Seligman *et al.*, 1968). Two alternative enzyme detection systems, developed particularly for use in double immunostaining procedures, are those based on glucose oxidase (Campbell & Bhatnagar, 1976) and alkaline phosphatase (Mason & Sammons, 1978). The enzyme glucose oxidase is obtained from *Aspergillus niger* and, like peroxidase, can be incorporated into a third layer complex with biotin and avidin. The chromogen in this case is a coloured, insoluble formazan, which arises from the oxidation of glucose and the concomitant reduction of a tetrazolium salt. There are a number of different tetrazolium salts that produce formazans of different colours (Altman, 1976). A particular advantage of using this enzyme is that it is not present in mammalian tissues and therefore a step to block endogenous enzyme activity is not needed.

Alkaline phosphatase is an enzyme generally isolated from calf intestine and like the other two enzymes can be incorporated into the ABC procedure. The development process for this enzyme is based on either the reduction of tetrazolium salts or on the production of coloured diazo compounds. The colours of the end-product diazo compounds are dependent on the pH of the incubation medium, with alkali media resulting in blue deposits and acid media producing red compounds.

Both of these enzyme techniques are widely used, particularly for double immunostaining, but neither of them is as sensitive as the peroxidase-based system. The stain deposits produced tend to be fairly coarse and they are no match for horseradish peroxidase in terms of morphological definition (De Jong, Van Kessel-Van Vark & Rapp, 1985).

Chromogen enhancements

Enhancement techniques are particularly useful when only routinely fixed tissue is available and consequently antigen presentation is low. There are a number of different techniques available (see review by Scopsi & Larsson, 1986). Intensification of DAB staining product can take place during the standard development incubation, e.g. with imidazole (Straus, 1982), cobalt chloride (Hsu & Soban, 1982) or nickel ammonium sulphate (Shu, Ju & Fan, 1988) or after this, e.g. silver methenamine (Rodríguez *et al.*, 1984) or ferric ferricyanide (Nemes, 1987). The heavy metal intensifications can sometimes suffer with problems of enhanced background staining and therefore require very accurate incubation times. This is not always possible when large numbers of sections are being processed in parallel.

A further method for intensifying the immunostaining obtained with the ABC method is to sequentially incubate sections with additional avidin–biotin complex solutions, which results in an increased deposition of horseradish peroxidase and hence increased sensitivity (Cattoretti et al., 1988). This is also useful because it allows higher dilutions of primary antisera to be used.

In addition to the techniques mentioned above, a number of other steps can be tried to improve the quality of immunostaining. These include prolongation of incubation times (Brandtzaeg, 1981), and repetition of primary (Gu, Islam & Polak, 1983) or second- and third-layer antisera (Vacca, 1982). Assuming the antibody being used is specific for the antigen being sought, background staining is generally due to weak interactions (hydrophobic or electrostatic) between antibodies and tissue components. This can be reduced by increasing the dilution of the primary antiserum, treating with unrelated IgG or washing with detergent. However, be careful that such treatments do not alter the antigen–antibody interaction being studied.

Specificity controls

The basic principle underlying all immunocytochemical procedures is the specificity of the antibody–antigen reaction. For this reason it is essential that the specificity of immunostaining is verified. Antisera raised against a particular peptide may crossreact with structurally related peptides that have homologies in their amino acid sequences (Ju et al., 1986; Williams et al., 1987). This problem can be largely overcome by the preabsorption of the antiserum with its purified antigen prior to immunostaining (Petrusz et al., 1976, 1977; Swaab, Pool & Van Leeuwen, 1977; Larsson, 1983). This involves incubating the primary antiserum with its antigen for 16 h at 4 °C before it is applied to the tissue section. The antiserum should be maximally diluted to conserve stocks of antigen, which is often very expensive and hence in short supply. If the normal antiserum produces positive immunostaining while the preabsorbed antiserum gives a negative result, this would suggest that the antiserum is indeed specific for that antigen. The specificity of the antiserum can be further characterized by preabsorption with related antigens that are known to be present in the tissue of interest. Generally an antigen concentration of $1–10$ nmol ml^{-1} of optimally diluted antiserum is more than enough to abolish peptide immunostaining (Van Noorden, 1986).

Specificity tests are often run in conjunction with Western blotting analysis of tissue extracts, to help to confirm that the antigen of interest is actually present in the tissue being studied.

In the absence of the appropriate antigen for preabsorption studies, a number of other control experiments can be carried out to determine the specificity of the antibody being used. The extent of non-specific background staining can be determined by omitting the primary antiserum or one of the subsequent layers in order to produce a negative method control. Positive tissue controls should also be carried out to confirm the viability of the method. Non-specific background staining can be reduced by preincubating the sections with a solution of hydrogen peroxide in water or methanol (particularly for cryostat sections), which saturates any endogenous peroxidase activity. Background can be further reduced by adding normal serum from the donor species of the secondary antibody to the primary antibody diluent. This saturates sites in the tissue that might otherwise interact non-specifically with the secondary antiserum. Alternatively, it can be applied as a separate preincubation step.

Multiple staining

Multiple or sequential immunocytochemical procedures can be used to demonstrate two or more antigens simultaneously. Double fluorescent preparations are particularly effective because the different fluorophores can be viewed either separately or simultaneously depending on the microscope filter combinations used. If this method is not sensitive enough for the antigens of interest, multiple enzymatic methods can be employed. However, with enzymatic methods there is a danger of cross-reaction between the primary antibody used in the first set of reactions and the second antibody of the second set. Therefore, it is essential to use non-cross-reacting antibodies. An alternative method is to elute sections with acid after visualizing the first antigen to leave an insoluble reaction product in the tissue. The second antigen is then developed using a different enzyme marker (Nakane, 1968). If the antigens of interest are known to be localized in different tissue compartments, sequential enzymatic stains can be used without elution as long as the DAB from the first set of reactions is enhanced in some way that allows it to be distinguished from that in the second.

Another alternative is to use thin serial or mirror-image sections (Gibson *et al.*, 1984) to co-localize antigens. If the sections are thin enough, some labelled cells will appear in adjacent sections. Mirror-image sections may be problematic if the tissue is very homogeneous and has no obvious landmarks to allow the alignment of sections.

Quantitative immunocytochemistry

Immunocytochemistry is an extremely versatile technique with numerous potential applications in both diagnostic and research medicine. One application of particular interest in our own work on human neurodegenerative diseases is the development of quantitative pathology. Until recently the interpretation of pathological specimens has essentially been regarded as a qualitative technique with the extraction of meaningful results dependent on the expertise of a trained observer, the pathologist. However, human nature being what it is, different observers will not always reach the same conclusions about what they are seeing and this may lead to wide variations in interpretation. Whilst the human eye and brain are extremely good at recognizing patterns within a field of view, they are less capable of producing quantitative data from a complex image. This can cause problems when setting general criteria for the diagnosis of a disease, e.g. Alzheimer's disease, that is based on the quantitative assessment of individual lesions in tissue sections. There is therefore an ever-increasing need for more rigorous and less subjective procedures that will allow the extraction of reliable quantitative data.

Staying with the example of Alzheimer's disease, we have previously shown that immunocytochemistry has a number of distinct advantages over other pathological procedures for quantitative analysis (Gentleman et al., 1989a). The staining is of high contrast and specificity (Figure 5.2) and is readily repeatable, which makes it ideal for computer image analysis and the subsequent production of reliable quantitative data. Such techniques can be used to improve diagnostic criteria and may play an important role in helping to determine the pathogenic mechanisms underlying the disease (Gentleman et al., 1992). For further information concerning the rapidly expanding field of quantitative pathology see Chapter 11.

Appendix: Immunostaining protocol

 (i) Mount cryostat/wax sections on PLL-coated slides and air dry at room temperature.
 (ii) Dehydrate sections through graded alcohols to xylene (or less hazardous equivalent).
 (iii) Block endogenous peroxidase by immersion in 0.3% (v/v) hydrogen peroxide in methanol for 30 min at room temperature.
 (iv) Rehydrate sections through graded alcohols to distilled water.
 (v) Incubate sections with primary antisera in a humid atmosphere at 4 °C for 16 h. Antisera diluted in phosphate buffered saline (PBS) containing 0.01% (w/v) sodium azide, 0.25% (v/v) Triton X-100 and 3% (v/v) normal serum.
 (vi) Rinse in three changes of PBS, 5 min each change.
 (vii) Incubate in biotinylated goat anti-rabbit IgG (for rabbit polyclonals) or biotinylated horse anti-mouse IgG (for mouse monoclonals) diluted in PBS containing 0.25% (v/v) Triton X-100 (1:100), for 45–60 min at room temperature.
 (viii) Rinse in three changes of PBS, 5 min each change.
 (ix) Incubate sections with non-immune avidin–biotin complex diluted in PBS containing 0.25% (v/v) Triton X-100 (1:200) for 45–60 min at room temperature.
 (x) Rinse in two changes of PBS, 5 min each change.
 (xi) Wash twice in 0.1 M acetate buffer, 10 min each change.

(xii) Immerse in developing solution* for 5–10 min.

(xiii) Wash in running tap water, dehydrate through graded alcohols, clear in xylene and mount.

*Glucose oxidase–DAB–nickel developing solution

(After Shu, Ju & Fan, 1988)

(a) Dissolve 2.5 g of nickel ammonium sulphate in 50 ml of 0.2 M sodium acetate buffer (pH 6.0).

(b) Dissolve 50–60 mg of DAB in 50 ml of distilled water.

Solution (a) and solution (b) are mixed immediately before use and then 200 mg β-D-glucose, 40 mg of ammonium chloride and 1–1.5 mg of glucose oxidase are added to the mixture.

References

Altman, F. P. (1976). Tetrazolium salts and formazans. *Progress in Histochemistry and Cytochemistry*, **9**, 1–56.

Berod, A., Hartman, B. K. & Pujol, J. F. (1981). Importance of fixation in immunohistochemistry: use of formaldehyde solutions at variable pH for the localization of tyrosine hydroxylase. *Journal of Histochemistry and Cytochemistry*, **29**, 844–50.

Brandtzaeg, P. (1981). Prolonged incubation staining of immunoglobulins and epithelial components in ethanol and formaldehyde fixed paraffin-embedded tissues. *Journal of Histochemistry and Cytochemistry*, **29**, 1302–15.

Campbell, G. T. & Bhatnagar, A. S. (1976). Simultaneous visualization by light microscopy of two pituitary hormones in a single tissue section using a combination of indirect immunohistochemical methods. *Journal of Histochemistry and Cytochemistry*, **24**, 448–52.

Cattoretti, G., Berti, E., Schiro, R. *et al*. (1988). Improved avidin-biotin-peroxidase complex (ABC) staining. *Histochemical Journal*, **20**, 75–80.

Coons, A. H., Creech, H. J. & Jones, R. N. (1941). Immunological properties of an antibody containing a fluorescent group. *Proceedings of the Society of Experimental Biology and Medicine*, **47**, 200–2.

Coons, A. H., Leduc, E. H. & Connolly, J. M. (1955). Studies on antibody production. I. A method for the histochemical demonstration of specific antibody and its application to a study of the hyperimmune rabbit. *Journal of Experimental Medicine*, **102**, 49–60.

De Jong, A. S. H., Van Kessel-Van Vark, M. & Rapp, A. K. (1985). Sensitivity of various visualisation methods for peroxidase and alkaline phosphatase activity in immunoenzyme-histochemistry. *Histochemical Journal*, **17**, 1119–30.

De Mey, J., Hacker, G. W., De Waele, M. & Springall, D. R. (1986). Gold probes in light microscopy. In *Immunocytochemistry. Modern methods and applications*, 2nd edn (ed. J. M. Polak & S. Van Noorden), pp. 71–88. Wright & Sons, Bristol.

De Mey, J. & Moeremans, M. (1986). Raising and testing polyclonal antibodies for immunocytochemistry. In *Immunocytochemistry. Modern methods and applications*, 2nd edn (ed. J. M. Polak & S. Van Noorden), pp. 3–12. Wright & Sons, Bristol.

Gentleman, S. M., Allsop, D., Bruton, C. J. *et al.* (1992). Quantitative differences in the deposition of β/A4 protein in the sulci and gyri of frontal and temporal isocortex in Alzheimer's disease. *Neuroscience Letters*, **136**, 27–30.

Gentleman, S. M., Bruton, C., Allsop, D. *et al.* (1989a). A demonstration of the advantages of immunostaining in the quantification of amyloid plaque deposits. *Histochemistry*, **92**, 355–8.

Gentleman, S. M., Falkai, P., Bogerts, B. *et al.* (1989b). Distribution of galanin-like immunoreactivity in the human brain. *Brain Research*, **505**, 311–15.

Gibson, S. J., Polak, J. M., Bloom, S. R. *et al.* (1984). Calcitonin gene-related peptide immunoreactivity in the spinal cord of man and of eight other species. *Journal of Neuroscience*, **4**, 3101–11.

Graham, R. C. & Karnovsky, M. J. (1966). The early stages of absorption of injected horseradish peroxidase in the proximal tubules of mouse kidney: ultrastructural cytochemistry by a new technique. *Journal of Histochemistry and Cytochemistry*, **14**, 291–303.

Gu, J., Islam, K. K. & Polak, J. M. (1983). Repeated application of first layer antiserum improves immunostaining, a modification of indirect immunofluorescence procedure. *Histochemical Journal*, **15**, 475–83.

Harrison, P. J., Proctor, A. W., Barton, A. J. *et al.* (1991). Terminal coma affects messenger RNA detection in post mortem human temporal cortex. *Molecular Brain Research*, **9**, 161–4.

Hartman, B. K., Zide, D. & Adenfriend, S. A. (1972). The use of dopamine-β-hydroxylase as a marker for the central noradrenergic nervous system in the rat brain. *Proceedings of the National Academy of Sciences, USA*, **69**, 2722–6.

Holgate, C. S., Jackson, P., Cowen, P. N. & Bird, C. C. (1983). Immunogold-silver staining: new method of immunostaining with enhanced sensitivity. *Journal of Histochemistry and Cytochemistry*, **31**, 938–44.

Hsu, S. M., Raine, L. & Fanger, H. (1981). Use of avidin–biotin–peroxidase complex (ABC) in immunoperoxidase technique. *Journal of Histochemistry and Cytochemistry*, **29**, 577–80.

Hsu, S. M. & Soban, E. (1982). Color modification of diaminobenzidine (DAB) precipitation by metallic ions and its application to double immunohistochemistry. *Journal of Histochemistry and Cytochemistry*, **30**, 1079–82.

Huang, W.-M., Gibson, S. J., Facer, P. *et al.* (1983). Improved adhesion for immunocytochemistry using high-molecular weight polymers of L-lysine as a slide coating. *Histochemistry*, **77**, 275–9.

Huang, S. N., Minassian, H. & More, J. D. (1976). Application of immunofluorescent staining on paraffin sections improved by trypsin digestion. *Laboratory Investigation*, **35**, 383–90.

Ju, G., Hökfelt, T., Fischer, J. A. *et al.* (1986). Does cholecystokinin-like immunoreactivity in primary sensory neurones represent calcitonin gene-related peptide? *Neuroscience Letters*, **68**, 305–10.

Kitamoto, T., Ogomori, K., Tateishi, J. & Prusiner, S. B. (1987). Formic acid pretreatment enhances immunostaining of cerebral and systemic amyloids. *Laboratory Investigation*, **57**, 230–6.

Köhler, G. & Milstein, C. (1976). Continuous cultures of fused cells producing antibodies of predefined specificity. *Nature*, **256**, 495–7.

Larsson, L. I. (1983). Methods for immunocytochemistry of neurohormonal peptides. In *Handbook of chemical neuroanatomy, Vol 1, Methods in chemical neuroanatomy* (ed. A. Björklund & T. Hokfelt), pp. 147–209. Elsevier Biomedical Press, Amsterdam & New York.

Mason, D. Y. & Sammons, R. E. (1978). Alkaline phosphatase and peroxidase for double immunoenzymatic labelling of cellular constituents. *Journal of Clinical Pathology*, **31**, 454–62.

McLean, I. W. & Nakane, P. K. (1974). Periodate-lysine-paraformaldehyde fixative. A new fixation for immunoelectron microscopy. *Journal of Histochemistry and Cytochemistry*, **22**, 1077–83.

Nakane, P. K. (1968). Simultaneous localisation of multiple tissue antigens using the peroxidase-labeled antibody method: a study in pituitary glands of the rat. *Journal of Histochemistry and Cytochemistry*, **16**, 557–60.

Nakane, P. K. & Pierce, G. B. (Jr) (1966). Enzyme labelled antibodies: preparation and application for the localisation of antigen. *Journal of Histochemistry and Cytochemistry*, **14**, 929–31.

Nemes, Z. (1987). Intensification of 3,3′-diaminobenzidine precipitation using the ferric ferricyanide reaction, and its application in the double-immunoperoxidase technique. *Histochemistry*, **86**, 415–19.

Palay, S. L., McGee-Russel, S. M., Gordon, S. & Grille, M. A. (1962). Fixation of neural tissues for electron microscopy by perfusion with solutions of osmium tetroxide. *Journal of Cell Biology*, **12**, 385–410.

Petrusz, P., Sar, M., Ordonneau, P. & Di Meo, P. (1976). Specificity in immunocytochemical staining. *Journal of Histochemistry and Cytochemistry*, **24**, 1110–12.

Petrusz, P., Sar, M., Ordonneau, P. & Di Meo, P. (1977). Can specificity ever be proved in immunocytochemical staining? *Journal of Histochemistry and Cytochemistry*, **25**, 390–1.

Polak, J. M. & Van Noorden, S. (eds.) (1986). *Immunocytochemistry. Modern methods and applications*, 2nd edn. Wright & Sons, Bristol.

Ritter, M. A. (1986). Raising and testing of monoclonal antibodies for immunocytochemistry. In *Immunocytochemistry. Modern methods and applications*, 2nd edn (ed. J. M. Polak & S. Van Noorden), pp. 13–25. Wright & Sons, Bristol.

Rodríguez, E. M., Yulis, R., Peruzzo, B. *et al.* (1984). Standardization of various applications of methacrylate embedding and silver methenamine for light and electron microscopy immunocytochemistry. *Histochemistry*, **81**, 253–63.

Scopsi, L & Larsson, L. I. (1986). Increased sensitivity in peroxidase immunocytochemistry. A comparative study of a number of peroxidase visualization methods employing a model system. *Histochemistry*, **84**, 221–30.

Seligman, A. M., Karnovsky, M. J., Wasserkrug, H. L. & Hanker, J. S. (1968). Non-droplet ultrastructural demonstration of cytochrome oxidase activity with a polymerizing osmiophilic reagent, diaminobenzidine (DAB). *Journal of Cell Biology*, **38**, 1–14.

Shu, S., Ju, G. & Fan, L. (1988). The glucose oxidase-DAB-nickel method in peroxidase histochemistry of the nervous system. *Neuroscience Letters*, . **85**, 169–71.

Sloviter, R. S. & Nilaver, G. (1987). Immunocytochemical localization of GABA-, cholecystokinin-, vasoactive intestinal polypeptide-, and somatostatin-like immunoreactivity in the area dentata and hippocampus of the rat. *Journal of Comparative Neurology*, **256**, 42–60.

Springall, D. R., Hacker, G. W., Grimelius, L. & Polak, J. M. (1984). The potential of the immunogold-silver staining method for paraffin sections. *Histochemistry*, **81**, 603–8.

Sternberger, L. A. (1979). *Immunocytochemisty*, 2nd edn. Wiley, New York.

Straus, W. (1982). Imidazole increases the sensitivity of the cytochemical reaction for peroxidase with diaminobenzidene at a neutral pH. *Journal of Histochemistry and Cytochemistry*, **30**, 491–3.

Swaab, D. F., Pool, C. W. & Van Leeuwen, F. W. (1977). Can specificity ever be proved in immunocytochemical staining? *Journal of Histochemistry and Cytochemistry*, **25**, 388–90.

Vacca, L. L. (1982). 'Double bridge' techniques of immunocytochemistry. In *Techniques in Immunocytochemistry*, Vol. 1 (ed. G. R. Bullock & P. Petrusz), pp. 152–82. Academic Press, New York & London.

Van Noorden, S. (1986). Tissue preparation and immunostaining techniques for light microscopy. In *Immunocytochemistry. Modern methods and applications*, 2nd edn (ed. J. M. Polak & S. Van Noorden), pp. 26–53. Wright & Sons, Bristol.

Williams, R. G., Dimaline, R., Varro, A. *et al.* (1987). Cholecystokinin octapeptide in rat central nervous system. Immunocytochemical studies using a monoclonal antibody that does not react with CGRP. *Neurochemistry International*, **11**, 433–42.

6

Autoradiography in brain research: theory, practice and applications

M. CLAIRE ROYSTON

Introduction

The technique of autoradiography has been extensively utilized within the fields of biomedical and neuroscience research. Over 7000 papers were published between the years of 1988 and 1991, in which it was the principal research tool. Applied to the field of brain research this powerful technique is now being used to investigate the detailed neurochemical anatomy of the brain. These studies have increased our knowledge and understanding of the normal distribution of transmitters and their associated receptors in the brain. From this rapidly expanding database, investigations are now beginning to determine if specific abnormalities of neurotransmitter systems underlie the dysfunctioning of the brain in both neurodegenerative conditions, such as Parkinson's disease, and neurodevelopmental disorders, such as Down's syndrome or schizophrenia.

Autoradiography may be defined as 'the visualization, on photographic emulsion, of the distribution of radiation that originates from radioactive material incorporated into a specimen or section of tissue'. Essentially, the tissue absorbs and scatters the radiation so that the resultant image reflects the distribution of radioactivity in the specimen and its modification by the structures of the specimen. By utilizing a ligand with a specific affinity for a particular tissue component, e.g. a receptor sub-type or re-uptake site, radiation is 'introduced' specifically into the particular aspect of the tissue specimen that is to be studied. Measurement of the bound radioactivity can then be used as an index or marker of the tissue component under study.

Autoradiography can be performed at the macroscopic level, e.g. whole body autoradiography to reveal the distribution of radioactivity through the various tissues and organs of a whole animal. Autoradiography at the light microscope level uses smaller grain size photographic emulsions to yield a greater resolution and the pattern of radioactivity can be quantitatively assessed within discrete structures visible at the light microscopic level, e.g. basal ganglia. Track autoradiography uses photographic film with a thicker coating of emulsion and the passage of β-particles can be recognized at the microscopic level by the characteristic path they 'carve' through the emulsion. Finally, autoradiography has been utilized at the electron microscopic level to visualize the distribution of radioactivity within structures only visible at this higher level of resolution, e.g. the synapse.

The alternative, and complementary, 2-deoxyglucose technique, utilizes similar principles but provides a more dynamic picture of the brain's activity. The technique was developed by Sokolov *et al.* (1977) and provides a graphic representation of glucose consumption under both normal and abnormal experimental conditions. It has been suggested that changes in regional 2-deoxyglucose uptake resulting from experimental manipulations, e.g. administration of a drug, are a direct consequence of changes in synaptic activity during the period of uptake (Schwartz *et al.*, 1979).

Theoretical basis

The historical development of autoradiography as a biological technique has been outlined by Rogers (1979), beginning with the demonstration of the uptake of radioactive iodine by the thyroid gland, which was followed by the preparation of autoradiographs showing the distribution of the radio-iodine in the gland. Prior to the development of liquid emulsions, the latent image was visualized by placing the section in direct contact with a lantern plate. The use of liquid emulsions was a significant advance and markedly increased the resolution of the autoradiographic image. These early studies relied upon the *in vivo* introduction of the radioligand to the intact animal; this is clearly limited by a number of practical constraints, the most important of which is the relative impenetrability of the blood–brain barrier. This problem was overcome with the introduction of *in vitro* autoradiographic techniques (Young and Kuhar, 1979), which avoid the necessity of giving the live animal a radioligand and have been particularly useful in studies establishing the details of receptor localization. *In vitro* autoradiography also has the important advantage of allowing studies to be performed on human post-mortem material.

The theoretical basis of autoradiography has a number of facets, which will be examined in turn. This chapter focuses on the two techniques that have been most widely used to study the brain: *in vitro* autoradiography and the 2-deoxyglucose technique.

Photographic emulsion

A crystalline lattice of silver bromide forms the basis of the photographic emulsion used in autoradiography. A small input of energy (5 eV) is necessary to cause the movement of free electrons within this lattice, leading to the deposition of silver within the crystal. This property is fundamental to the formation of the latent image on the emulsion. In an idealized situation, this energy is supplied solely by the ionizing radiation incorporated into the specimen. However, the reaction is not specific and silver deposition can result from exposure of the emulsion to light, mechanical pressure, thermal excitation and other reducing chemicals. These factors account for the 'background' image and are discussed in detail later in the chapter.

The emulsion used in autoradiography has three characteristics that govern the quality/usefulness of the resultant image:

> sensitivity
> resolution
> definition

The sensitivity of the film is determined by the composition of the photographic emulsion. The silver bromide crystals are held in a supporting medium of gelatine; the higher the ratio of silver bromide to gelatine the greater the sensitivity of the film. Sensitivity is also increased by having a minimal distance between the emulsion and the specimen and techniques to ensure this intimate contact, e.g. absence of an anti-scratch coating on the film or mechanisms for holding the specimen in direct apposition to the film, will increase sensitivity. The resolution of the image is most critically determined by the size of the silver bromide crystals formed within the lattice. Resolution is increased if a large number of small crystal complexes occur. There are then more possibilities for crystals to be activated or not so that events occurring within the emulsion will be reproduced with a greater accuracy or resolution. However, the smaller the mean diameter of the silver bromide crystals in an emulsion the more difficult it becomes to achieve a high sensitivity. This is because a very small crystal can only contain a correspondingly small component of the trajectory of the free electron, so that the total energy liberated within the crystal by the particle is correspondingly small. Thus, there is a theoretical balance between the physical demands of an emulsion to achieve a high sensitivity and those necessary for maximal resolution.

Definition is a simpler concept and relates to the contrast between exposed and unexposed areas of film. Thus, this is determined by the characteristics of the base onto which the emulsion is coated to produce the film. An ideal base would therefore be both clear and colourless.

Radioligands

These studies all depend on the binding of a radioactive compound – radioligand – to the receptor site to be studied. Thus the first prerequisite is the availability of a specific radioligand labelled to a known specific activity that is stable and has a high affinity for the receptor under study. Many such radioligands have been extensively researched and are now available commercially. The binding of the radioligand to a receptor follows the standard kinetics very similar to those of the classic enzyme–substrate interaction and the Scatchard equation can be derived (see Bennett & Yamamura, 1985, for details), which describes the interaction of a receptor with a ligand:

$$B/F = (B_{max} - B)/K_d$$

Thus, knowing the concentration of radioligand bound (B) and free (F) at equilibrium allows the determination of the affinity of the receptor (K_d) and the maximum number of binding sites (B_{max}). When we are interpreting the results of a study we wish to be able to equate an alteration (decrease or increase) in binding as reflecting an alteration in number or affinity of a receptor. To make this interpretation with certainty the specificity of the radioligand:receptor binding must be established, i.e. the radioligand binds to the receptor and no other site. This feature should be assessed prior to carrying out an experiment; an ideal radioligand binds with high affinity, low capacity, forms a stable complex and follows similar drug competition profiles to those established for the receptor.

Essentially all radioligands that are available possess an affinity to bind nonspecifically to both biological and nonbiological material (e.g. test tubes, filters, etc.). Clearly this property will be a confounding variable. For many receptors, drugs with structures markedly different from the radioligand are available, which interact potently at the receptor site. The parallel experiment includes an excess concentration of these drugs to define the non-specific binding. The specific binding can then be calculated as

Specific = Total − Non-specific

In principle, radioisotopes emitting α, β or γ radiation can be utilized in autoradiography. In practice, many experiments utilize β-emitting radioisotopes for several reasons. Firstly, available nuclear emulsions have a very high efficiency for β-particles, particularly those with low energies. Secondly, many of the elements of biological interest have suitable β-emitting isotopes – ^{3}H, ^{14}C, ^{35}S and ^{125}I. Tritium is the isotope most often used in studies of the autoradiographic localization of receptor distributions. The β-particles emitted by tritium have a very low energy (18.6 keV), so that the images produced on the photographic film arise only from emissions originating very near ($< 5\ \mu$m) the tissue surface (Rogers, 1979). This has the advantage of producing a high resolution image and that variation in the thickness of sections does not affect the density of the autoradiographic image. However, using tritium has several disadvantages compared to other isotopes, including the long exposure times required. Tritium emissions are attenuated and quenched to different degrees, depending on the chemical composition of the tissue containing the tritium.

Development of the latent image

The latent image is correctly defined in a statistical manner (Meas and James, 1966) as 'any exposure-induced changes that increase the development probability from < 0.5 to > 0.5 under a specified set of development conditions'. More simply the effect of radiation on the photographic emulsion causes a *latent image* representing the deposition of silver molecules, which are then visualized by the development process. Thus, the final image obtained is critically dependent upon the chemical processes that constitute the developmental process. Altering the developmental process will change that population of 'exposed' crystals that will be converted to developed silver grains and thereby visualized. A number of factors directly affect the development process and must therefore be carefully controlled in an experiment if valid comparisons of images are to be made.

Background

Ideally, the radiation incorporated into the tissue specimen should be the sole source of radiation and therefore responsible for the development of all silver grains. However, silver grains that are not from radiation of the source appear on all autoradiographs, and constitute the background. This has two important consequences: firstly, the level of background determines the minimum level of radioactivity that can be reliably detected. Secondly, in order to make meaningful comparisons between tissue sections the variability in the amount of background must be minimized. The important causes of background silver grains are:

    exposure to light
    mechanical pressure
    contamination of the emulsion with reducing agents
    environmental radiation
    spontaneous appearance
    thermal excitation

Obvious simple precautions will help to minimize the amount of background. These include safe-light working conditions whenever film is being handled, careful construction of autoradiographic cassettes that ensures even pressure is applied to the film, clean working conditions to avoid contamination and, finally, films should be incubated in a temperature-controlled environment.

Summary

The essential feature of autoradiography is that it allows the distribution of radioactivity to be related to the structure of the specimen. Each silver bromide molecule within the photographic emulsion is essentially acting as an individual detector system, hence detailed information about level isotope binding across a structure, e.g. the cortex, can be revealed. Therefore, autoradiography gives information concerning both *amount* and *distribution pattern* within a structure. This contrasts with other techniques such as, for example, detection by scintillation counting of the amount of bound radioisotope within a homogenate tissue preparation. Thus, by utilizing radioisotopes incorporated into ligands having an affinity for specific neuronal uptake or receptor sites, information concerning specific neurotransmitters can be obtained at an anatomical level.

2-Deoxyglucose studies

This technique rests on three basic tenets:

1. There is a direct relationship between the functional *activity* of the brain and its energy *consumption*.
2. Glucose is the major energy source of the brain.
3. 2-Deoxyglucose is taken up and phosphorylated by brain cells in an identical manner to glucose, but cannot be further metabolized and therefore accumulates within the cell.

In a experiment, a set 'load' of 2-deoxyglucose is introduced into the experimental animal and then the blood concentration of 2-deoxyglucose monitored. Standard equations describing the kinetics of 2-deoxyglucose in both the monkey and rat have been established (Sokolov, 1981). The animal is subsequently sacrificed and the levels of 2-deoxyglucose that have accumulated in the target tissue are assessed autoradiographically. These values and the blood concentration of 2-deoxyglucose over the time span of the experiment can be used to calculate the rates of glucose utilization within the target tissue. These values can then be used as a direct index of the level of functioning of the target tissue. Many experiments establish base-line values in the first part of the study and in the second part introduce a drug or other intervention postulated to directly affect the functioning of the tissue under study. Direct comparison of values in the first and second parts of the experiment allow inferences to be drawn of the effect of the drug or intervention on the functioning of the target tissue.

Practical steps

The practical section of this chapter will concentrate on the commonest technique – *in vitro* autoradiography. Whilst many comments are also applicable to the preparation of autoradiographs in 2-deoxyglucose studies, the reader is referred to more specialized texts for detailed descriptions of this technique (Sokolov *et al.*, 1977). Undertaking an *in vitro* autoradiographic experiment can be broken down into four basic steps:

preparation of sections
incubation with radioligand
development of autoradiographic image
obtaining results

Each step raises a number of methodological points, which will be dealt with in the following sections.

Preparation of sections

The quality of the final autoradiographic image is directly determined by the processing and storage of the fresh brain tissue, preparation of the section and handling of the section during the experimental procedure, and exposure to film. A variety of approaches to the initial processing and storage of tissue have been used by investigators and are largely determined by practical constraints. The overriding aim is to have as short a post-mortem delay as possible. For animal experiments the time the animal is sacrificed can be predetermined by the experimenter and material can be immediately frozen. In human brain research this is not possible and post-mortem delays of 12–15 h are the practical minimum that can be achieved. Therefore, investigations of the stability of the neurochemical parameter to be studied should be established prior to undertaking an autoradiographic experiment.

Rapid freezing of the brain material is necessary to avoid ice crystals forming within the material, which will produce artefacts in the final autoradiographic image. This can be achieved by using a freezing liquid such as isopentane or liquid nitrogen or by placing small pieces of material on dry ice until the material is completely frozen. The technique chosen depends largely on what is readily available. The larger the block of material to be frozen the more difficult it is to achieve rapid freezing of the whole block. Experience has shown that it is very difficult to achieve 'snap-freezing' of anything larger than approximately 20 cm^3. Therefore, a dissection procedure must frequently be employed to subdivide the brain into manageable-sized blocks. A detailed protocol must be established in order to ensure that precisely comparable blocks are produced from each subject in an experiment.

Prepared snap-frozen blocks are then stored at $-70\,°C$ in air-tight sealed bags. Blocks exposed to the air whilst being stored rapidly develop a feature analogous to the 'freezer burn' of food that is stored unwrapped in a domestic freezer. Essentially, the surface of the block becomes dehydrated resulting in extensive tissue damage. In order to prevent this, each block should be wrapped in film to exclude the air and stored in small individual plastic bags. Stored in this manner the blocks can be stored for up to 2 years before sections are prepared.

When all the blocks for a given experiment are available, frozen sections can be prepared. It is important to note that although frozen sections can be stored in a $-70\,°C$ freezer, once cut the sections will deteriorate, again mostly due to dehydration. Hence sections should be cut and used in an experiment as quickly as possible. As a working rule of thumb, sections have a freezer life of 2–3 weeks before appreciable tissue deterioration begins.

Ultra-thin sections are not required if using a β-emitting isotope, since the low energy of these particles allow them to penetrate only up to 5 μm tissue depth. Therefore, since there is no advantage to thin sections, the technically easier to prepare thicker section (20 or 30 μm) can be used.

The glass slides for an experiment should be carefully prepared, as significant background binding to the slide can occur if poorly prepared or dirty slides are used. New glass slides should be washed twice in distilled water and then dipped in dilute nitric acid, followed by a further two washes in distilled water. Slides should then be dried in a dust-free environment. A gelatine-based subbing solution is used to coat the slides and slowly dried in a warm oven and stored in sealed bags at -4 °C until use.

After sections are cut and thaw-mounted onto the prepared slides, the main difficulty is avoiding condensation from forming on the surface of the section. One way of avoiding this is to dry each slide on a warm plate and then immediately place the slides in the freezer in racks, storing the sections in an anhydrous environment.

Incubation with radioligand

The details of this stage will be dictated by the optimum binding conditions of the radioligand used in a particular study. However, there are a number of features common to the majority of protocols. A pre-incubation stage in a suitable biological buffer solution is often included, as this helps to reduce the level of non-specific binding. Sections are then incubated with the radioligand and parallel incubations set up with a displacing agent, in order to determine the non-specific binding. Autoradiographic images representing both *total* and *non-specific* binding can then be produced, thereby allowing the calculation of the levels of *specific* binding.

During the incubation process, the main practical problem is evaporation, resulting in some portions of sections drying out and the pooling of ligand over other portions of the section. It is therefore helpful to incubate sections in trays lined with buffer-soaked filters to provide a saturated atmosphere, thereby reducing the evaporation process.

The final stage is to stop the incubation process by dipping the slide into ice-cold buffer solution and then washing each section – to remove unbound ligand – by taking each slide through a series of 10 s washes and finally a 1 s wash in ice-cold distilled water. The sections can then be air-dried prior to apposing each slide to photographic film. The optimum length of exposure time should be determined for a given tissue and radioligand. Films are placed in light-tight cassettes, where it is important to ensure that an even pressure is applied across all the slides to avoid artefactual effects caused by pressure differences.

If quantitative analysis of results is to be undertaken, then radioactive standards should be exposed to each sheet of film used. Commercially produced radioactive standards are available, alternatively brain paste standards incorporating a known amount of radioactivity can be prepared and used in the same manner.

Development of autoradiographic image

As has been previously discussed, there are a number of factors that will affect the developmental process and these must be standardized within an experimental if valid comparisons between images are to be made. A detailed protocol standardizing the following should therefore be established:

concentration, pH, temperature of developing agent
length of time each film is placed in the developing agent
degree of agitation of the developing solution
use of an acidic 'stop-bath' to rapidly terminate the development reaction

The undeveloped silver bromide can then be solubilized in a fixing solution and washed out of the gelatine in running water.

Obtaining results

The autoradiographic image comprises silver grains held in the gelatine medium. In essence, the more bound radioligand the greater the energy input into the emulsion and the greater the number of silver molecules deposited and the 'darker' the latent image subsequently revealed as dark areas on the autoradiograph. Similarly, a small amount of bound radioligand results in pale areas on the final autoradiograph. Several features of the emulsion response can be quantified and compared. Three main features have been used:

counting of silver grains
track number
optical density

Counting silver grains

The simplest feature of the emulsion to quantify is the number of silver grains and early methods of quantification were based on counting the number of developed silver grains in a defined area. This was both time-consuming and prone to counting errors. It is important to note that the relationship between incident energy and number of silver grains is a logarithmic one; this means that, at high radiation doses, detail in the image may become lost as a single silver ion can only respond once, even if it is excited several times. In addition, if the density of developed silver grains becomes very high, then it becomes increasingly difficult to identify and count individual silver grains.

Track counting

A similar approach is to count the number of 'tracks' that have been carved through the emulsion as excited electrons move through it. This technique is very precise – there is no difficulty relating grain density to radioactive disintegrations, since each track simply represents an individual β-particle. However, it has the major drawback that identifying the track is very labour intensive and images have to be examined at a high level of magnification to allow the tracks to be identified, making it difficult to relate the information to the specimen as a whole.

Optical density

The third feature of the emulsion that can be readily quantified is the optical density. The developed silver grains reduce the transparency of the film, i.e. the proportion of incident light that is transmitted through the film. Optical density is defined as log (1/Transparency). This may readily be examined using computerized image analysis techniques. A video camera attached to the microscope of macro-lens systems is used to input an image of the autoradiograph to a digitizing tablet. Providing that the incident light source is stable, measurements of the optical density of defined areas within the image can then be readily made.

Calibration of the autoradiographs

A major advance in the quantification of information from autoradiographs was the introduction in 1981 of calibrated radioactive standards that were co-exposed with the tissue sections under study (Unnerstall *et al.*, 1981). Autoradiographic microscales consist of layers of radioactive colourless polymer arranged in order of increasing specific activity. For each assay a set of these calibrated microscales are cut, at the same thickness as the sections, and exposed and developed alongside the sections. Thus, optical densities can be converted into molar quantities of receptor-bound radioligand by comparing the optical density of the tissue sample to the known standard.

In plotting a standard curve there are two pertinent factors: the response of the video camera is related in a non-linear manner to luminant intensity of light (Gonzalez & Wintz, 1977) and the response of the film to radioactive decay is also non-linear and follows a complex sigmoidal curve (Ehn & Larsson, 1979; Young & Kuhar, 1979). It is therefore important to examine the manufacturer's specification of the camera used in the image analysis system and, if necessary, adjustments made to compensate for a non-linear camera response. Some newer cameras on the market have additionally been modified to increase the reliability of optical density measurements. These cameras are provided with an internal 'black reference', allowing them to re-set themselves to the same black standard at the beginning of every line scan (1500 s^{-1}).

A number of alternative approaches have been developed to account for the complex response pattern of the film to radioactivity. In a review of this issue, Miller, Hoffer & Zahniser (1988) suggested that a logistic function curve fit will not only provide a good fit to the data, but in addition allow the determination of the existence of deviant points in the standards by the goodness of fit to the standard curve.

As has been described, optical density measurement refers to the amount of light absorbed by the sample. In film autoradiography the sample necessarily lies on film and it is standard practice to assume that the light absorbed by the film is a constant.

Two types of measurements can therefore be made:

amount of radioligand binding in a given structure
pattern of the distribution of radioligand within the structure

The assessment of the amount of binding in a structure is a simple procedure in which each structure is outlined planimetrically on the digitized image and the average optical density within the defined boundaries computed. This is a reliable technique for relatively large structures with a simple profile, e.g. amygdala or caudate nucleus, but is prone to considerable error if complex structures are to be outlined. In addition, for small objects there is considerable error on the measurement owing to the edge artefact. Eilbert, Gallistel & McEachron (1990) studied this problem by analysing data compiled from many outlines drawn by several investigators, concluding that the variation in their results constituted a major source of error. They suggested that multiple outlining and a consistent set of outlining criteria should be developed and used in order to minimize this error.

The pattern of binding within a structure presents a more difficult problem. For example, the cortex is subdivided into laminae both anatomically and functionally. The pattern of distribution on receptors across the cortex is therefore of interest. Again the problem arises of the reliable identification of boundaries between the cortical laminae on the autoradiograph. Accurate identification is difficult and introduces the type of error discussed above. Moreover, the laminae are only reliably identified on histologically stained sections; transferring this information accurately to the autoradiograph is problematic and a further potent source of bias. A possible approach to avoiding this problem has been developed (Royston *et al.*, 1991), where only the pial surface and the white matter interface need to be defined, rather than all the inter-laminar boundaries.

Practical applications

The main prerequisite for an autoradiographic study is to have a sensible question to ask. Autoradiography is a relatively expensive and time-consuming technique and many experiments have failed because there is no clear plan from the outset of what information is required from the autoradiographs that have been carefully prepared. The following studies illustrate the types of questions that autoradiography has been used to investigate.

Mapping studies

Following the development of the *in vitro* autoradiography technique it was extensively used in this type of study, for example Rakic, Goldman-Rakic & Gallagher (1988) examined the binding properties and distribution pattern of nine neurotransmitter receptors and their sub-types in the visual cortex. These studies were undertaken as part of an extensive programme of research on the visual cortex. They found that the visual cortical areas differed in density and lamination of neurotransmitter receptors and suggested that this may be reflected in the differing sensitivity to circulating levels of neurotransmitters and pharmacologically active compounds underlying cortical mechanisms.

As new radioligands have become available, mapping studies have continued to provide valuable information. Csillag *et al.* (1987) determined the regional distribution of the three major sub-types of opioid binding sites in the brains of 1-day-old chicks. Reviewing their findings in relation to the functioning of the brain, they suggested that the greatest density of opiate receptor binding sites coincide with regions involved in higher order sensory processing and memory storage.

A further example of the type of information that can be obtained from mapping studies is illustrated in a study by Persson *et al.* (1991). Benzodiaze-pine receptor binding was studied in whole human brain cryosections, including saturation experiments to determine the binding characteristics. This information can then be used to supply vital information that can be incorporated into studies using *in vivo* scanning techniques (positron emission tomography), concerning the positioning of the scanner and indicating significant regions of interest to be studied.

Developmental studies

Autoradiographic studies examining material from fetal, neonatal and adult subjects have demonstrated age-dependent changes in a number of neurotrans-mitters, for example 5-HT$_2$ (Gross-Isseroff *et al.*, 1990), excitatory amino acids (Slater, McConnell & D'Souza, 1992). In many of these types of study (e.g. Bar-Peled *et al.*, 1991, studying 5-HT$_{1A}$ receptors) prenatal peaks of the density of receptors have been demonstrated leading to the important suggestion that these receptors play a role in human brain development.

Neuropsychiatric studies

Following on from the findings of both mapping studies and developmental studies, attention is increasingly focused on using autoradiography to study post-mortem brain samples from neuropsychiatric studies. Often these studies are 'driven' by neuropathological studies indicating abnormalities in a particular area and the prevalent neurotransmitters of that area are then examined. Studies suggesting neuropathological abnormalities within the hippocampal formation have been followed up by studies of glutamate binding sites within this area. Kerwin, Patel & Meldrum (1990) have demonstrated a loss of kainate receptor subtype within the CA_4/CA_3 region of the hippocampus in schizophrenic compared with control subjects. Moreover, an *in situ* hybridization study examining the messenger RNA encoding the kainate receptor has shown a 70% reduction in this area in schizophrenia (Harrison, McLaughlin & Kerwin, 1991). These studies reflect the possible importance of glutamate in the pathophysiology of schizophrenia.

2-Deoxyglucose studies

The 2-deoxyglucose technique has been used to elucidate the neural mechanisms underlying the motor symptoms of parkinsonism. In the study by Mitchell *et al.* (1989) a specific and profound decrease in 2-deoxyglucose uptake was demonstrated within the subthalamic nucleus, leading to the suggestion that this nucleus plays a pivotal role in the mechanism of the parkinsonian symptoms and opens up the possibility of therapeutic approaches that are not restricted to an action in the striatum.

Summary

This chapter has tackled autoradiography at three levels, theory, practice and application, which have been illustrated with recent studies utilizing the technique to answer the types of questions currently being investigated in relation to the human brain. Autoradiography is helping us to elucidate in detail the abnormalities of neurotransmitters that underlie the dysfunctioning of the brain in a range of both degenerative and neurodevelopmental conditions. From a greater understanding of the neural mechanisms underpinning these conditions it is hoped that more specific and effective treatment strategies can be developed.

References

Bar-Peled, O., Gross-Isseroff, R., Ben-Hur, H. *et al.* (1991). Fetal human brain exhibits a prenatal peak in the density of serotonin 5-HT$_{1A}$ receptors. *Neuroscience Letters*, **127**, 173–6.

Bennett, J. P. & Yamamura, H. I. (1985). Neurotransmitter receptor binding. In *Neurotransmitters, hormone or drug receptor binding methods*, 2nd edn. (ed. H. I. Yamamura), pp. 61–89. Raven Press, New York.

Csillag, A., Bourne, R. C., Kalman, M. *et al.* (1987). Opioid receptor binding sites in the chick brain: a quantitative autoradiographic study. *Neuroscience*, **22**, 5303.

Ehn, E. & Larsson, B. (1979). Properties of an anti-scratch layer-free X-ray film for the autoradiographic registration of tritium. *Scientific Tools*, **26**, 24–9.

Eilbert, J. L., Gallistel, C. R. & McEachron, D. L. (1990). The variation in user drawn outlines on digital images: effects on quantitative autoradiography. *Computerised Medical Imaging and Graphics*, **14**, 331–9.

Gonzalez, R. C. & Wintz, P. W. (1977). *Digital image processing*. Addison-Wesley, Reading.

Gross-Isseroff, R., Salama, D., Israli, M. & Biegon, A. (1990). Autoradiographic analysis of age dependent changes in serotonin 5-HT$_2$ receptors of the human brain postmortem. *Brain Research*, **519**, 223–7.

Harrison, P. J., McLaughlin, D. & Kerwin, R. W. (1991). Decreased hippocampal expression of a glutamate receptor gene in schizophrenia. *Lancet*, **337**, 450–2.

Kerwin, R., Patel, S. & Meldrum, B. (1990). Quantitative autoradiographic analysis of glutamate binding sites in normal and schizophrenic brain postmortem. *Neuroscience*, **39**, 25–32.

Miller, J. A., Hoffer, B. J. & Zahniser, N. R. (1988). An improved calibration procedure for computer-based quantitative autoradiography utilizing a mathematical model for the non linear response of camera and film. *Journal of Neuroscience Methods*, **22**, 233–8.

Mitchell, I. J., Clarke, C. E., Boyce, S. *et al.* (1989). Neural mechanisms underlying parkinsonian symptoms based upon regional uptake of 2-deoxyglucose in monkeys exposed to 1-methyl-4-phenyl-1,2,3,6 tetrahydropyridine. *Neuroscience*, **32**, 213–26.

Persson, A., d'Argy, R., Gillberg, P. G. *et al.* (1991). Autoradiography with saturation experiments of ^{11}C-Ro 15-1788 binding to human brain sections. *Journal of Neuroscience Methods*, **36**, 53–61.

Rakic, P., Goldman-Rakic, P. S. & Gallagher, D. (1988). Quantitative autoradiography of major neurotransmitter receptors in the monkey striate and extrastriate cortex. *Journal of Neuroscience*, **8**, 3670–90.

Rogers, A. W. (1979). *Techniques of autoradiography*. Elsevier, Amsterdam.

Royston, M. C., Slater, P., Simpson, M. D. C. & Deakin, J. F. W. (1991). Analysis of laminar distribution of kappa opiate receptors in human cortex: comparison between schizophrenic and normal. *Journal of Neuroscience Methods*, **36**, 145–53.

Schwartz, W. J., Smith, C. B., Davidsen, L. *et al.* (1979). Metabolic mapping of functional activity in the hypothalamo neurohypophysial system of the rat. *Science*, **205**, 723–5.

Slater, P., McConnell, S. & D'Souza, S. W. (1992). Age-related changes in binding to excitatory amino acid uptake sites in temporal cortex in human brain. *Developmental Brain Research*, **65**, 157–60.

Sokolov, L. (1981). Localization of functional activity in the central nervous system by measurement of glucose utilization with radioactive deoxyglucose. *Journal of Cerebral Blood Flow Metabolism*, **1**, 7–36.

Sokolov, L., Reivich, M., Kennedy, C. *et al.* (1977). The ^{14}C-deoxyglucose method for the measurement of local cerebral glucose utilization: theory, procedure and normal values in the conscious and anaesthetized albino rat. *Journal of Neurochemistry*, **28**, 897–916.

Unnerstall, J. R., Kuhar, M. J., Niehoff, D. L. & Palacios, J. M. (1981). Benzodiazepine receptors are coupled to a sub-population of gamma-aminobutyric acid (GABA) receptors: evidence from a quantitative autoradiographic study. *Journal of Pharmacology and Experimental Therapeutics*, **218**, 797–804.

Young, W. S. & Kuhar, M. J. (1979). A new method for receptor autoradiography: ^{3}H-opioid receptors in rat brain. *Brain Research*, **179**, 255–270.

PART 2

Applications

7

Human prion diseases

MARK S. PALMER and JOHN COLLINGE

Introduction

Like many other neurological disorders, prion disorders can occur in an inherited familial context or as sporadic diseases (Prusiner, 1991). However, they are unique in that they are also transmissible, either by inoculation of experimental animals or, rarely, by direct contact with affected tissues or their derivatives. The infectious agent in these diseases has been called a 'prion' and is believed by many to consist principally of an abnormal, disease-related isoform of a protein known as the prion protein, PrP (Prusiner, 1982). The normal cellular isoform of PrP (PrP^C) is a phosphatidylinositol anchored membrane-bound glycoprotein found on the surface of neurones and other cells of the body (Stahl et al., 1987). PrP^C is rapidly turned over, while the abnormal form found in disease, PrP^{Sc}, accumulates intracellularly (Taraboulos, Serban & Prusiner, 1990) and may be deposited as amyloid in plaques. PrP^{Sc} is unusual in its remarkable resistance to degradation by proteases. Although PrP^C is expressed early in development (Manson et al., 1992) recent observations on mice in which the prion protein gene has been ablated suggest that the protein is not necessary for normal development (Büeler et al., 1992) and its function remains unknown.

The human prion diseases encompass Creutzfeldt–Jakob disease (CJD), Gerstmann–Sträussler–Scheinker syndrome (GSS) and kuru. Kuru is a transmissible disease, now virtually extinct, that reached epidemic proportions amongst certain tribes in Papua New Guinea due to ritualistic cannibalism. CJD is recognized clinically by the occurrence of a rapidly progressive dementia with myoclonus and is often accompanied by pyramidal signs, cerebellar ataxia or extrapyramidal features. The clinical course of the disease is rapid and death usually follows within 12 months of onset. GSS patients present with a chronic cerebellar ataxia, and dementia occurs later in the clinical course. The disease is of longer duration than CJD. Clinical onset is usually in the third to fourth decade and the duration of illness is about 5 years, although there are recorded cases of up to 11 years duration. Confirmation of prion disease requires the neuropathological demonstration of spongiosis affecting any part of the cerebral grey matter, neuronal loss and proliferation and hypertrophy of astrocytes (Beck & Daniel, 1987). These changes are sometimes accompanied by the accumulation of partially protease-resistant amyloid plaques. About 15% of all cases are familial, while GSS is nearly always described in a familial context, both cases showing an autosomal dominant pattern of segregation. In addition to the sporadic and familial forms of CJD, a few cases world-wide have been recognized to derive from iatrogenic causes.

Prion protein

Attempts to purify infectious agent from affected brains have always resulted in a fraction whose predominant macromolecular component is PrP^{Sc}. PrP^{Sc} cannot be dissociated from infectivity and accumulating evidence suggests that it is the principal component of the infectious agent in these diseases. Human PrP is a protein of 253 amino acids (254 in hamster and mouse) (Figure 7.1). The amino terminus contains a 22 amino acid signal sequence, which is cleaved during synthesis in the endoplasmic reticulum. The carboxy terminal also contains a signal sequence of 23 amino acids, which is cleaved on addition of a glycosylinositol phospholipid anchor (Stahl *et al.*, 1987, 1990*a*, *b*). An internal disulphide bond forms a loop in the molecule within which are attached two asparagine-linked oligosaccharides.

Treatment of PrP^{Sc} with proteinase-K results in the loss of 67 amino acids from the N-terminus of the mature PrP^{Sc}, leaving a 141 amino acid proteinase-K resistant core. This core has a relative molecular mass of 27–30 kD and is called PrP27–30. The region that is cleaved from PrP^{Sc} contains an interesting set of repeated sequences. Two repeats of GG(S/N)RYP(Q/P)QG overlap with a longer set of five repeats, P(H/Q)GGG-(-/T)WGQ. The significance of these repeats is unknown, although they are highly conserved amongst all species sequenced so far. These repeats possess a high degree of β structure but are unnecessary for the amyloid properties of PrP polymers as they are absent from PrP27–30, which retains infectivity. A short stretch between residues 96

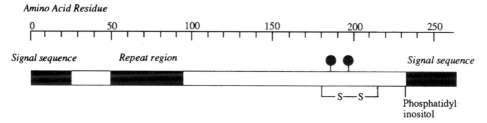

Figure 7.1. Representation of the prion protein amino acid sequence. The signal sequences are cleaved during maturation. The resulting carboxy-terminal end is then modified by addition of a phosphatidylinositol. The location of an internal disulphide bond is indicated by S–S. The locations of the two *N*-linked oligosaccharides are indicated by black circles.

and 112 contains a domain controlling the topology of PrP in artificial membrane, and is designated the stop transfer effector (Lopez *et al.*, 1990; Yost *et al.*, 1990).

The gene for PrP (*PRNP*) is located on the short arm of chromosome 20, in a region syntenic with the region of mouse chromosome 2 that encodes murine PrP (Liao *et al.*, 1986; Robakis *et al.*, 1986; Sparkes *et al.*, 1986). It is constitutively expressed in the adult brain though it is regulated during development. PrP mRNA and choline acetyltransferase increase in parallel in the septum during development, whereas PrP expression occurs earlier in other brain regions (Mobley *et al.*, 1988). The highest levels of PrP mRNA expression are found in neurones (Kretzschmar *et al.*, 1986).

Following the identification of the human PrP gene it was possible to look for linkage of familial cases to markers flanking PrP or to identify mutations in the PrP gene. Hsiao *et al.* demonstrated linkage between the PrP gene and GSS in two families (Hsiao *et al.*, 1989). Affected members of these families contained a missense mutation in codon 102. The demonstration of linkage was the first formal proof that GSS was a genetic disease. However, although all other mammalian PrP open reading frames that have been sequenced encode proline at the equivalent position, it remained a possibility that proline–leucine substitution at codon 102 would be a benign, though uncommon, polymorphism that was in genetic linkage with the actual disease locus. The subsequent demonstration of this mutation co-segregating with disease in other GSS kindreds in Germany, US and Japan, as well as in the original kindred reported by Gerstmann (Kretzschmar *et al.*, 1991), and its absence from all control populations that have been looked at, strongly indicate that the mutation is indeed pathogenic. To investigate further the pathogenicity of the leucine substitution at codon 102, Hsiao *et al.* created transgenic mice in which mutant PrP genes were introduced, containing a leucine-encoding codon at the equivalent position in mouse PrP (Hsiao *et al.*, 1990). These mice, expressing both normal mouse PrP and murine-PrP^{Leu}, spontaneously developed a neurological disease. Although only detected at low levels, PrP^{Sc} was present in the brains of the spontaneously sick mice and it has now proved possible to transmit the disease from these affected mice to unaffected ones (Hsiao *et al.*, 1992*b*). This experiment very clearly shows that not only is the leucine 102 mutation pathogenic, but that the generation of abnormal PrP can follow from an alteration in the primary structure of PrP^{C} in the absence of exposure to infectious agents.

Another mutation in the PrP open reading frame had been previously reported in the UK in a family with CJD (Collinge *et al.*, 1989; Owen *et al.*, 1989). This proved to be an insertion of 144 base pairs in the region encoding the octapeptide motif representing six extra octapeptide repeats (Figure 7.2). This insertion was subsequently found in five additional families in a screening of over 100 cases of neurodegenerative disease. In none of the five reference cases had the previous clinical diagnosis included CJD or GSS. Diagnoses

Wild Type Allele

CCT	CAg	GGC	GGT	GGT	GGC	TGG	GGG	CAG	R1
Pro	Gln	Gly	Gly	Gly	Gly	Trp	Gly	Gln	
CCT	CAT	-	GGT	GGT	GGC	TGG	GGG	CAG	R2
Pro	His	-	Gly	Gly	Gly	Trp	Gly	Gln	
CCT	CAT	-	GGT	GGT	GGC	TGG	GGG	CAG	R2
Pro	His	-	Gly	Gly	Gly	Trp	Gly	Gln	
CCc	CAT	-	GGT	GGT	GGC	TGG	GGa	CAG	R3
Pro	His	-	Gly	Gly	Gly	Trp	Gly	Gln	
CCT	CAT	-	GGT	GGT	GGC	TGG	GGt	CAa	R4
Pro	His	-	Gly	Gly	Gly	Trp	Gly	Gln	

Allele with Insertion

CCT	CAg	GGC	GGT	GGT	GGC	TGG	GGG	CAG	R1
Pro	Gln	Gly	Gly	Gly	Gly	Trp	Gly	Gln	
CCT	CAT	-	GGT	GGT	GGC	TGG	GGG	CAG	R2
Pro	His	-	Gly	Gly	Gly	Trp	Gly	Gln	
CCT	CAT	-	GGT	GGT	GGC	TGG	GGG	CAG	R2
Pro	His	-	Gly	Gly	Gly	Trp	Gly	Gln	
CCT	CAT	-	GGT	GGT	GGC	TGG	GGG	CAG	R2
Pro	His	-	Gly	Gly	Gly	Trp	Gly	Gln	
CCc	CAT	-	GGT	GGT	GGC	TGG	GGa	CAG	R3
Pro	His	-	Gly	Gly	Gly	Trp	Gly	Gln	
CCT	CAT	-	GGT	GGT	GGC	TGG	GGG	CAG	R2
Pro	His	-	Gly	Gly	Gly	Trp	Gly	Gln	
CCc	CAT	-	GGT	GGT	GGC	TGG	GGG	CAG	R3´
Pro	His	-	Gly	Gly	Gly	Trp	Gly	Gln	
CCT	CAT	-	GGT	GGT	GGC	TGG	GGG	CAG	R2
Pro	His	-	Gly	Gly	Gly	Trp	Gly	Gln	
CCT	CAT	-	GGT	GGT	GGC	TGG	GGG	CAG	R2
Pro	His	-	Gly	Gly	Gly	Trp	Gly	Gln	
CCc	CAT	-	GGT	GGT	GGC	TGG	GGa	CAG	R3
Pro	His	-	Gly	Gly	Gly	Trp	Gly	Gln	
CCT	CAT	-	GGT	GGT	GGC	TGG	GGt	CAa	R4
Pro	His	-	Gly	Gly	Gly	Trp	Gly	Gln	

Figure 7.2. Comparison of the repeat region in the wild type allele with the sequence in those individuals with a 144 bp insertion equivalent to six extra repeats.

included Alzheimer's disease, Huntington's disease, Pick's disease and familial presenile dementia. Genealogical work established that all of the families were in fact part of the same pedigree (Poulter *et al.*, 1992). This pedigree, spanning seven generations, contains 47 affected family members on whom information has been collected. This pedigree demonstrated considerable heterogeneity in both the clinical presentation and neuropathological features of individuals (Collinge *et al.*, 1992), all of whom have the same mutations in the prion protein gene. An individual who died in the 1940s had a rapid clinical course with a reported duration of 6 months, and was described as having Heidenhahn's variant of CJD. Pathologically, there was gross status spongiosis and astrocytosis affecting the entire cerebral cortex, and histology from this case was used to illustrate classic CJD pathology in Greenfield's *Neuropathology* textbook. By contrast, there are other family members with much longer duration of illness, more typical of GSS (4–8 years), with only mild and subtle spongiform change, insufficient for a morphological diagnosis of CJD, and a case from this family had none of the characteristic features of spongiform encephalopathy. Since there is a significant degree of variability in both the clinical presentation and neuropathological findings within this family, it is clear that terms such as Creutzfeldt–Jakob disease, Gerstmann–Sträussler syndrome and spongiform encephalopathy are less useful in describing these cases, although each retains its own specific meaning within the broader spectrum.

The recognition of pathogenic mutations in the prion gene means that there is now a simple diagnostic test for the prion diseases, namely the sequencing of the PrP gene in likely patients. This has been applied to a number of individuals and about a dozen mutations and polymorphisms have now been identified (Figure 7.3). The next section will look at each of these mutations in turn and will present details of the clinical phenotype associated with each one.

PrP mutations

Insertions

Additional insertions in the region of PrP that consists of a repeated octapeptide motif have been reported in the past year. The 144 base pair insertion described above represents an insertion of six extra octapeptide repeats. Goldfarb *et al.* report familial CJD cases associated with five, seven and eight extra octapeptides in the open reading frame (Goldfarb *et al.*, 1991*a*). Material from each of these families has been transmitted to primates. Detailed clinical descriptions of the family with seven extra repeats have been presented elsewhere (Brown *et al.*, 1992*b*). Members of this family have an early-onset disease with very protracted duration (one case was still living after 13 years). The neuropathology ranges from marked spongiform change, gliosis and

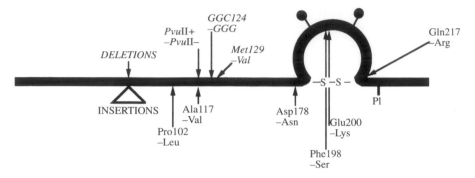

Figure 7.3. Location of the mutations and polymorphisms within the prion protein. The numbering is the same as in Figure 7.1, codon and amino acid residues having the same number. Mutations are in bold, polymorphisms are in lighter italic. The location of the phosphatidylinositol anchor, disulphide bond and glycosylation sites are indicated.

neuronal loss in the proband to a mild gliosis and neuronal loss with no spongiform change in her affected daughter with similar duration of disease (11 and 10 years respectively). In addition, there is a report of an affected individual with a nine-repeat insertion (Owen *et al.*, 1992).

Point mutations

PrP-Leu^{102}

Unrelated families from France, Germany, UK, US and Japan have been found with this mutation, as well as the original family, described by Gerstmann, which came from Austria. There is considerable variation in clinical and neuropathological presentation, which can include ataxia, amnesia and disorientation with spinocerebellar signs (Doh-ura *et al.*, 1989; Hsiao *et al.*, 1989).

PrP-Val^{117}

Codon 117 is associated with two nucleotide changes. One is a non-coding third base change which is found in about 2.5% of the population (Palmer & Collinge, unpublished data) and is therefore a harmless polymorphism. It can be easily detected as it destroys a Pvu II restriction site in the open reading frame (Wu *et al.*, 1987). The other change is a coding mutation changing an alanine to valine. This was first described in a French family (Doh-ura *et al.*, 1989) and subsequently in a US family of German origin (Hsiao *et al.*, 1991*a*). The US family was originally described as having familial Alzheimer's disease, but was reclassified to GSS upon finding PrP-immunostaining amyloid plaques. The family had pre-senile dementia with extrapyramidal signs. The French family had pre-senile dementia with pyramidal and pseudobulbar features, with cerebellar signs in some family members.

PrP-Asn[178]

A mutation at codon 178 was first described in 1991 (Goldfarb *et al.*, 1991*b*). There have been a number of reports recently that discuss the clinical phenotype associated with this mutation in a number of families (Goldfarb, Brown & Gajdusek, 1992*a*). The mutation has been reported to be associated with an early age of onset (fourth decade) and prolonged illness (up to 5 years) and absence of periodic EEG activity (Brown *et al.*, 1992*a*). The disease almost always presents with an insidious loss of memory (Brown *et al.*, 1991). Neuropathology shows a diversity in the intensity and topography of spongiform change, gliosis and neuronal loss. While the cerebellum is rarely involved, irrespective of the clinical picture, the cerebral cortex and nuclei of the caudate and basal ganglia are most seriously involved. Pathology is, however, quite variable and while members of a French family (Wui) with this mutation have necrotic white matter demyelination, four members of an American family had minimal or absent neuropathology. Plaques were absent in all cases. An affected member of the Wui family has been described with a distinct clinical phenotype (Laplanche *et al.*, 1992). This patient had a late onset disease (57 years of age) and presented with memory loss, vertigo and disorientation, which progressed over the next 9 months to the classical characteristics of CJD, dementia, myoclonus and periodic EEG activity.

That the phenotype associated with the 178 mutation is highly variable and is probably affected by many other genetic factors is highlighted by the demonstration of this mutation in patients presenting with fatal familial insomnia (FFI) (Medori *et al.*, 1992*b*). FFI was first described in 1986 as a rapidly progressing familial disease, with a mean age of onset of 49 and duration of 13 months, characterized clinically by untreatable insomnia, dysautonomia (which included hyperthermia, tachycardia, hypertension and hyperhydrosis) and motor signs, and neuropathologically by selective atrophy of the anterior ventral and medial thalamic nuclei (Lugaresi *et al.*, 1986). Because of the presence of various degrees of atrophy and reactive astrogliosis in other thalamic nuclei, together with spongiosis of the cerebellar cortex in one individual, it was appropriate to investigate the possibility of there being a mutation in the prion protein gene (Manetto *et al.*, 1992). The finding of a mutation at codon 178 highlights the power of genetic analysis in unravelling the aetiology of unusual neurological disorders (Medori *et al.*, 1992*a*). What remains to be determined is what factors are acting to give rise to distinct phenotypes in families with the same mutation. Analysis of the prion protein from the brains of affected individuals has shown that there is proteinase-K-resistant PrP present, though not in all members of every kindred. However, the size of the proteinase-resistant core of PrP^{Sc}, as determined by Western blot analysis, is different from that found in sporadic cases of CJD. It is not yet known how this compares to the size of protein in other codon 178 cases.

PrP-Ser[198]

Two recent papers have reported novel mutations in the PrP open reading frame in patients with an atypical from of GSS. Both mutations occur in families in which affected individuals have been shown to have neurofibrillary tangles (NFTs) like those of Alzheimer's disease. The first was reported in a large Indiana kindred (Dlouhy et al., 1992). This pedigree has been traced back to 1792 and clinical or historical examinations are available on affected members from each generation. All affected individuals have NFTs composed of paired helical filaments in the cerebral cortex and subcortical nuclei. In the cerebrum these coexist with uni- and multi-centric plaques as well as plaques of Alzheimer's type. The amyloid core of the plaques can be labelled with antibodies against PrP but not β-amyloid. Sequencing of affected patients has shown the presence of a mutation at codon 198 resulting in a phenylalanine to serine substitution. This mutation co-segregates with disease in this pedigree and generates a Lod score of over 6 at $\phi = 0$. As discussed later, this family also demonstrated the effect of methionine/valine heterozygosity at codon 129 on age of onset. The 198 mutation lies on an allele bearing valine at codon 129. Interestingly, an earlier report had looked at the amino acid sequence of the PrP fragment deposited in plaques from two of the affected members (Tagliavini et al., 1991). The fragment contained amino acids from residues 58 to about 150 so did not include the codon 198 mutation. However, in one of the individuals who is known to be heterozygous at codon 129 by genotyping, only the valine allele-derived protein fragment was found. This supports the hypothesis that the progression of disease might involve protein that is homologous to the mutant form (at least with respect to residue 129 – see below).

PrP-Arg[217]

The other family that was found to have neurofibrillary tangles and a PrP mutation was Swedish (Hsiao et al., 1992a). Affected individuals began to show symptoms of dementia at least 4 years before development of gait ataxia, dysphagia and confusion, which occurred in the few months preceding death. The mutation in this family was a glutamine to arginine substitution at residue 217. In addition to the new mutation a novel variation was found on the non-mutant allele in which there was a silent third-base C–G transversion at the glycine encoding codon 124. It remains to be seen to what extent either the 198 or 217 mutations may contribute towards the formation of NFTs, or whether there is a common pathway in neurodegeneration shared with Alzheimer's disease that leads to this processing.

PrP-Lys^{200}

This subtype was originally described in a Polish sibling pair with CJD (Goldgaber *et al.*, 1989). It accounts for ethnogeographic clustering of CJD in Slovakia, Libyan Jews in Israel, Sephardic Jews in Greece and familial CJD in Chile (Goldfarb *et al.*, 1992*b*). Two UK families have also been identified; one had Libyan Jewish ancestry but the other appears to be a separate UK focus (Collinge *et al.*, 1993). Patients with this subtype present with a rapidly progressive dementia, myoclonus and pyramidal, cerebellar or extra-pyramidal signs. There is a characteristic pseudoperiodic picture on EEG. The average age of onset for this disease is 55. Histologically these patients are typical of CJD, plaques are absent but PrP^{Sc} can be demonstrated by immunoblotting. This is the only PrP mutation so far that has been described in the homozygous state. Homozygosity did not affect the phenotype, as would be predicted for a dominant disorder (Hsiao *et al.*, 1991*b*). Also of interest is that a 78-year-old woman with this mutation has remained apparently asymptotic, suggesting that there is incomplete penetrance for the disease with this mutation.

Presymptomatic testing and counselling

The identification of PrP mutations in families with inherited prion disease allows a direct gene test for subjects at risk as well as providing accurate diagnosis in affected individuals. Such tests have already been carried out following careful genetic counselling. For counselling purposes, prion diseases are similar to Huntington's disease, for which protocols have been well established. Unlike Huntington's, however, for which there are many linked markers but no disease locus yet identified, the PrP gene test can be unambiguous as there is no possibility of recombination between the probe and the disease locus (Collinge *et al.*, 1991*b*). However, the possibility of incomplete penetrance, as seen in PrP-Lys^{200} disease, needs also to be included

Sporadic and iatrogenic CJD

Despite the advances in describing familial cases of CJD, there is still uncertainty as to the aetiology of the sporadic cases that account for about 85% of all CJD cases. In addition, there are a small number of cases that are known to have arisen by iatrogenic contamination. Such cases have arisen from the use of inadequately sterilized intracerebral electrodes, dura mater and corneal grafting, and from treatment with human cadaveric-derived pituitary growth hormone and gonadotrophin. In the UK, 1908 individuals received such growth hormone, each batch of which was prepared from a pool of over 3000 pituitaries, and six individuals have subsequently developed CJD (Buchanan, Preece & Milner, 1991). Each iatrogenic case received material from more than one batch and no single batch can be implicated in all cases. Most of the 1908 individuals receiving growth hormone probably were exposed to at least some of the contaminated material and it was possible to ask whether there was any evidence of genetic susceptibility amongst those who developed CJD. DNA from all six of the growth hormone cases and one gonadotrophin case was examined for sequence variation in the PrP gene. None of the known mutations were identified. However, there was a striking excess of homozygosity of the least frequent of two alternative amino acid residues at position 129. We found that four out of seven individuals were valine homozygous at position 129, compared with a normal frequency of 12% valine homozygosity, suggesting that valine homozygosity predisposes to iatrogenic susceptibility (Collinge, Palmer & Dryden, 1991*a*), at least for this source of contamination.

Sporadic cases of CJD are not thought to be due to environmental contamination, because of the uniform world-wide distribution of disease that only clusters in familial cases. However, it was possible to investigate whether or not there was evidence of genetic susceptibility or predisposition in sporadic cases in relation to the codon 129 polymorphism. Although there was no significant excess of valine homozygotes in a group of 22 confirmed sporadic cases, we did find that all but one of the cases were homozygous with respect to either methionine or valine (Palmer *et al.*, 1991). The single heterozygote was found on further enquiry to have a family history of dementia and was possibly not a sporadic case. This striking observation of homozygosity predisposing towards sporadic CJD provides support for a model of prion protein replication that has been proposed following observations in mice transgenic for the hamster prion protein gene (Prusiner *et al.*, 1990). This model is discussed in more detail below. A central component of the theory is that there is an interaction between PrP^{Sc} and PrP^{C} which results in the conversion of PrP^{C} into PrP^{Sc}, and that the interaction is facilitated by identity between the amino acid sequence of the two forms of the protein. Homozygotes, it is argued, would be more susceptible to the disease because of the identity of the protein sequences, leading to a more favourable interaction than in individuals who are heterozygous. Further evidence of the importance of the genotype at codon 129 comes from an observation of the extended pedigree with the 144 base pair insertion discussed above (Baker *et al.*, 1991, Poulter *et al.*, 1992, Collinge *et al.*, 1992). In this family all individuals with an early age of onset (under 40 years of age) were homozygous for the methionine allele (the mutation lies on this allele), while all those with a later age of onset were heterozygous. The phenomenon of early onset associated with homozygosity has also been demonstrated in the Indian kindred with codon 198 mutation, as mentioned above (Dlouhy *et al.*, 1992).

A protein model for prion diseases

How can a protein alone constitute an infective agent? No difference in primary sequence has been identified between the normal cellular isoform of

PrP (designated PrP^C) and the disease-related isoform (designated PrP^{Sc}). The difference between them is therefore assumed to reside in a post-translational change in PrP; protease resistant PrP^{Sc} is known to be derived from its protease sensitive precursor, PrP^C (Borcheldt *et al.*, 1990). It is hypothesized that the essential difference between PrP^{Sc} and PrP^C may be a conformational change and that the presence of a PrP^{Sc} molecule can catalyse this change in PrP^C, thus leading to a chain reaction of conformational change which itself constitutes the 'infective' process (Prusiner *et al.*, 1990). (Figure 7.4). According to such a model, PrP^C continues to be synthesized by the normal host cellular mechanisms and is then somehow converted to PrP^{Sc}, so that although novel, such a process of prion replication does not challenge fundamental biological principles. That some form of interaction between PrP molecules is involved in the disease process is suggested by work in transgenic mice which harbour normal hamster PrP transgenes (Prusiner *et al.*, 1990). While wild-type mice are usually not susceptible to infection with hamster prions (and the occasional

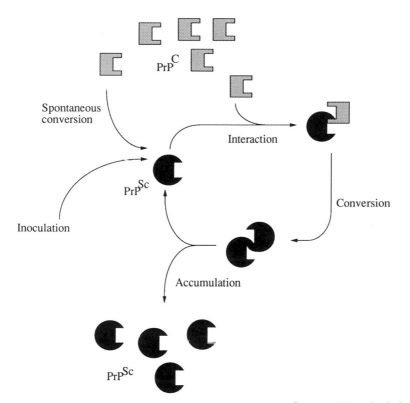

Figure 7.4. Model for the interaction of PrP^{Sc} and PrP^C. The light shaded squares represent PrP^C while the black circles represent PrP^{Sc}. The diagram indicates how PrP^{Sc}, arising by spontaneous conversion in sporadic or inherited cases, or by inoculation in iatrogenic cases, interacts with PrP^C and then catalyses the conversion of PrP^C into PrP^{Sc}. This leads to an accumulation of PrP^{Sc}, which further drives the cycle and leads to disease.

mouse that does succumb to infection does so after a prolonged incubation period), such transgenic mice expressing normal hamster PrP become fully susceptible to hamster-derived prions (Prusiner *et al.*, 1990). The so-called 'species barrier' to infection with prions was therefore abolished by introducing into these mice PrP obtained from the same species as the inoculum. Furthermore, if such transgenic mice, which express both normal murine PrP and normal hamster PrP, are inoculated with mouse-derived infective agent, the affected transgenic mice produce infective agent which is fully pathogenic for mice but not hamsters, while if these transgenic mice are inoculated with hamster-derived infective agent, the resulting affected transgenic mice produce infectivity fully pathogenic for normal hamsters and not mice. The idea that interaction between homologous PrP molecules is central to the disease process is further strengthened by the observation that sporadic CJD cases were predominately homozygotes with respect to the codon 129 mutation as discussed above.

Human prion diseases have inherited, sporadic and rare iatrogenic forms. According to the model discussed above, it is suggested that in the inherited forms of prion disease, prion protein with one of the known pathogenic mutations spontaneously undergoes the transformation to PrP^{Sc} (although this is still presumably an extremely rare event) and the disease-causing chain reaction of protein conformational change follows. The sporadic disease could then be accounted for by somatic mutation resulting in the formation of mutant PrP^{C} in a single cell and the line derived from it. The spontaneous transformation to PrP^{Sc} would occur as in inherited cases, the establishment and progression of disease occurring most easily in homozygotes (Palmer *et al.*, 1991). Iatrogenic disease, as in experimental disease following inoculation, arises when exogenous PrP^{Sc} is introduced and triggers formation of further PrP^{Sc}.

Conclusions

Despite their rarity, the inherited prion diseases are now arguably the best understood neurodegenerative disorders. It is now possible to make a DNA-based diagnosis of these conditions. The availability of a gene test, rather than a linked genetic marker as in Huntington's disease, enables precise pre-symptomatic (and antenatal) testing in families with one of the known mutations. In addition, it is possible to assign gene carriers to an early or late age of onset group, according to their homozygosity or heterozygosity at PrP codon 129 respectively, in a few of the inherited forms. It remains to be seen in how many types of inherited prion disease codon 129 genotype influences age of onset. Although codon 129 genotype influences age at onset it does not appear to affect the clinical features or pathology (Collinge *et al.*, 1992). Sporadic CJD cases heterozygous at codon 129 appear to have a longer duration illness and may account for 'atypical CJD' (Collinge & Palmer, 1991). PrP gene analysis performed on a routine blood sample should be considered in all cases of pre-senile dementia or ataxia. The apparent absence of a family history should not discourage analysis. It remains to be seen if a proportion of families currently categorized as other neurodegenerative disease will in fact turn out to have inherited prion diseases. The full range of phenotypic expression of inherited prion disease has still to be described but it is clear from the reports of fatal familial insomnia that the phenotypic range is already broader than that encompassed by the traditional spongiform encephalopathies.

Further research is needed to determine the nature of the post-translational modification that underlies the difference between PrP^C and PrP^{Sc}. According to the model of prion replication discussed above, ligands with selective binding properties for the disease-related isoform of PrP would be expected to interfere with the conversion of PrP^C to PrP^{Sc} and could result in the development of effective therapies for human prion diseases.

References

Baker, H. E., Poulter, M., Crow, T. J. *et al.* (1991). Aminoacid polymorphism in human prion protein and age at death in inherited prion disease. *Lancet*, **337**, 1286.

Beck, E. & Daniel, P. M. (1987). Neuropathology of transmissible spongiform encephalopathies. In *Prions: novel infectious pathogens causing scrapie and Creutzfeldt-Jakob disease* (ed. S. B. Prusiner & M. P. McKinley), pp. 331–85. Academic Press, San Diego.

Borcheldt, D. R., Scott, M., Taraboulos, A. *et al.* (1990). Scrapie and cellular prion proteins differ in their kinetics of synthesis and topology in cultured cells. *Journal of Cell Biology*, **110**, 743–52.

Brown, P., Goldfarb, L. G., Cathala, F. *et al.* (1991). The molecular genetics of familial Creutzfeldt–Jakob disease in France. *Journal of the Neurological Sciences*, **105**, 240–6.

Brown, P., Goldfarb, L. G., Kovanen, J. *et al.* (1992*a*). Phenotypic characteristics of familial Creutzfeldt–Jakob disease associated with the codon-178asn PRNP mutation. *Annals of Neurology*, **31**, 282–5.

Brown, P., Goldfarb, L. G., McCombie, W. R. *et al.*, (1992*b*). Atypical Creutzfeldt–Jakob disease in an American family with an insert mutation in the PRNP amyloid precursor gene. *Neurology*, **42**, 422–7.

Buchanan, C. R., Preece, M. A. & Milner, R. D. (1991). Mortality, neoplasia, and Creutzfeldt–Jakob disease in patients treated with human pituitary growth hormone in the United Kingdom. *British Medical Journal*, **302**, 824–8.

Büeler, H., Fischer, M., Lang, Y. *et al.* (1992). Normal development and behaviour of mice lacking the neuronal cell-surface PrP protein. *Nature*, **356**, 577–82.

Collinge, J., Brown, J., Hardy, J. *et al.* (1992). Inherited prion disease with 144 base pair gene insertion: II: clinical and pathological features. *Brain*, **115**, 687–710.

Collinge, J., Harding, A. E., Owen, F. *et al.* (1989). Diagnosis of Gerstmann–Sträussler syndrome in familial dementia with prion protein gene analyis. *Lancet*, **2**, 15–7.

Collinge, J. & Palmer, M. S. (1991). CJD discrepancy. *Nature*, **352**, 802.

Collinge, J., Palmer, M. S., Campbell, T. *et al.* (1993). Inherited prion disease (PRP lysine 200) in Britain; 2 case reports. *British Medical Journal*, **306**, 301–2.

Collinge, J., Palmer, M. S. & Dryden, A. J. (1991*a*). Genetic predisposition to iatrogenic Creutzfeldt–Jakob disease. *Lancet*, **337**, 1441–2.

Collinge, J., Poulter, M., Davis, M. B. *et al.* (1991*b*). Presymptomatic detection or exclusion of prion protein gene defects in families with inherited prion diseases. *American Journal of Human Genetics*, **49**, 1351–4.

Dlouhy, S. R., Hsiao, K., Farlow, M. R. *et al.* (1992). Linkage of the Indian kindred of Gerstmann–Sträussler–Scheinker disease to the prion protein gene. *Nature Genetics*, **1**, 64–7.

Doh-ura, K., Tateishi, J., Sasaki, H. *et al.* (1989). Pro-leu change at position 102 of prion protein is the most common but not the sole mutation related to Gerstmann–Sträussler syndrome. *Biochemical Biophysical Research Communications*, **163**, 974–9.

Goldfarb, L. G., Brown, P. & Gajdusek, D. C. (1992*a*). The molecular genetics of human transmissible spongiform encephalopathy. In *Prion diseases of humans and animals* (ed. S. B. Prusiner, J. Collinge, J. Powell & B. Anderton), pp. 00–00. Ellis Horwood, London.

Goldfarb, L. G., Brown, P., Haltia, M. *et al.* (1992*b*). Creutzfeldt–Jakob disease cosegregates with the codon 178-Asn PRNP mutation in families of European origin. *Annals of Neurology*, **31**, 274–81.

Goldfarb, L. G., Brown, P., McCombie, W. R. *et al.* (1991*a*). Transmissible familial Creutzfeldt–Jakob disease associated with five, seven, and eight extra octapeptide coding repeats in the PRNP gene. *Proceedings of the National Academy of Sciences, USA*, **88**, 10926–30.

Goldfarb, L. G., Haltia, M., Brown, P. *et al.* (1991*b*). New mutation in scrapie amyloid precursor gene (at codon 178) in Finnish Creutzfeldt–Jakob kindred. *Lancet*, **337**, 425.

Goldgaber, D., Goldfarb, L. G., Brown, P. *et al.* (1989). Mutations in familial Creutzfeldt–Jakob disease and Gerstmann–Straussler–Scheinker's syndrome. *Experimental Neurology*, **106**, 204–6.

Hsiao, K., Baker, H. F., Crow, T. J. *et al.* (1989). Linkage of a prion protein missense variant to Gerstmann–Straussler syndrome. *Nature*, **338**, 342–5.

Hsiao, K. K., Cass, C., Schellenberg, G. D. *et al.* (1991*a*). A prion protein variant in a family with the telencephalic form of Gerstmann–Sträussler–Scheinker syndrome. *Neurology*, **41**, 681–4.

Hsiao, K., Dlouhy, S. R., Farlow, M. R. *et al.* (1992*a*). Mutant prion proteins in Gerstmann–Sträussler–Scheinker disease with neurofibrillary tangles. *Neurology*, **1**, 68–71.

Hsiao, K. K., Groth, D., Scott, M. *et al.* (1992*b*). Genetic and transgenetic studies of prion proteins in Gerstmann–Sträussler–Scheinker disease. In *Prion disease of humans and animals* (ed. S. B. Prusiner, J. Collinge, J. Powell & B. Anderton), pp. 120–9. Ellis Horwood, London.

Hsiao, K., Meiner, Z., Kahana, E. *et al.* (1991*b*). Mutation of the prion protein in Libyan Jews with Creutzfeldt–Jakob disease. *New England Journal of Medicine*, **324**, 1091–7.

Hsiao, K. K., Scott, M., Foster, D. *et al.* (1990). Spontaneous neurodegeneration in transgenic mice with mutant prion protein. *Science*, **250**, 1587–90.

Kretzschmar, H. A., Honold, G., Seitelberger, F. *et al.* (1991). Prion protein mutation in family first reported by Gerstmann, Sträussler, and Scheinker. *Lancet*, **337**, 1160.

Kretzschmar, H. A., Prusiner, S. B., Stowring, L. E. & DeArmond, S. J. (1986). Scrapie prion proteins are synthesized in neurons. *American Journal of Pathology*, **122**, 1–5.

Laplanche, J. L., Chatelain, J., Thomas, S. *et al.* (1992). Uncommon phenotype for a codon 178 mutation of the human PrP gene. *Annals of Neurology*, **31**, 345.

Liao, Y. C., Lebo, R. V., Clawson, G. A. & Smuckler, E. A. (1986). Human prion protein cDNA: molecular cloning, chromosomal mapping, and biological implications. *Science*, **233**, 364–7.

Lopez, C. D., Yost, C. S., Prusiner, S. B. *et al*. (1990). Unusual topogenic sequence directs prion protein biogenesis. *Science*, **248**, 226–9.

Lugaresi, E., Medori, R., Baruzzi, P. M. *et al*. (1986). Fatal familial insomnia and dysautonomia, with selective degeneration of thalamic nuclei. *New England Journal of Medicine*, **315**, 997–1003.

Manetto, V., Medori, R., Cortelli, P. *et al*. (1992). Fatal familial insomnia: clinical and pathologic study of five new cases. *Neurology*, **42**, 312–19.

Manson, J., West, J. D., Thomson, V. *et al*. (1992). The prion protein: a role in mouse embryogenesis? *Development*, **115**, 117–22.

Medori, R., Montagna, P., Tritschler, H. J. *et al*. (1992*a*). Fatal familial insomnia: a second kindred with mutation of prion protein gene at codon 178. *Neurology*, **42**, 669–70.

Medori, R., Tritschler, H. J., LeBlanc, A. *et al*. (1992*b*). Fatal familial insomnia, a prion disease with a mutation at codon 178 of the prion protein gene. *New England Journal of Medicine*, **326**, 444–9.

Mobley, W. C., Neve, R. L., Prusiner, S. B. & McKinley, M. P. (1988). Nerve growth factor increases mRNA levels for the prion protein and the beta-amyloid protein precursor in developing hamster brain. *Proceedings of the National Academy of Sciences, USA*, **85**, 9811–5.

Owen, F., Poulter, M., Collinge, J. *et al*. (1992). A dementing illness associated with a novel insertion in the prion protein gene. *Molecular Brain Research*, **13**, 155–7.

Owen, F., Poulter, M., Lofthouse, R. *et al*. (1989). Insertion in prion protein gene in familial Creutzfeldt–Jakob disease. *Lancet*, **1**, 51–2.

Palmer, M. S., Dryden, A. J., Hughes, J. T. & Collinge, J. (1991). Homozygous prion protein genotype predisposes to sporadic Creutzfeldt–Jakob disease. *Nature*, **352**, 340–2.

Poulter, M., Baker, H. F., Frith, C. D. *et al*. (1992). Inherited prion disease with 144 base pair gene insertion. I: Genealogical and molecular studies. *Brain*, **115**, 675–85.

Prusiner, S. B. (1982). Novel proteinaceous infectious particles cause scrapie. *Science*, **216**, 136–44.

Prusiner, S. B. (1991). Molecular biology of prion diseases. *Sciences*, **252**, 1515–22.

Prusiner, S. B., Scott, M., Foster, D. *et al*. (1990). Transgenic studies implicate interactions between homologous PrP isoforms in scrapie prion replication. *Cell*, **63**, 673–86.

Robakis, N. K., Devine, G. E., Jenkins, E. C. *et al*. (1986). Localization of a human gene homologous to the PrP gene on the p arm of chromosome 20 and detection of PrP-related antigens in normal human brain. *Biochemical and Biophysical Research Communications*, **140**, 758–65.

Sparkes, R. S., Simon, M., Cohn, V. H. *et al*. (1986). Assignment of the human and mouse prion protein genes to homologous chromosomes. *Proceedings of the National Academy of Sciences, USA*, **83**, 7358–62.

Stahl, N., Baldwin, M. A., Burlingame, A. L. & Prusiner, S. B. (1990*a*). Identification of glycoinositol phospholipid linked and truncated forms of the scrapie prion protein. *Biochemistry*, **29**, 8879–84.

Stahl, N., Borchelt, D. R., Hsiao, K. & Prusiner, S. B. (1987). Scrapie prion protein contains a phosphatidylinositol glycolipid. *Cell*, **51**, 229–40.

Stahl, N., Borchelt, D. R. & Prusiner, S. B. (1990b). Differential release of cellular and scrapie prion proteins from cellular membranes by phosphatidylinositol-specific phospholipase C. *Biochemistry*, **29**, 5405–12.

Tagliavini, F., Prelli, F., Ghiso, J. *et al*. (1991). Amyloid protein of Gerstmann–Sträussler–Scheinker disease (Indiana kindred) is an 11 kd fragment of prion protein with an N-terminal glycine at codon 58. *EMBO Journal* **10**, 513–9.

Taraboulos, A., Serban, D. & Prusiner, S. B. (1990). Scrapie prion proteins accumulate in the cytoplasm of persistently infected cultured cells. *Journal of Cell Biology*, **110**, 2117–32.

Wu, Y., Brown, W. T., Robakis, N. K. *et al*. (1987). A PvuII RFLP detected in the human prion protein (PrP) gene. *Nucleic Acids Research*, **15**, 3191.

Yost, C. S., Lopez, C. D., Prusiner, S. B. *et al*. (1990). Non-hydrophobic extracytoplasmic determinant of stop transfer in the prion protein. *Nature*, **343**, 669–72.

8

Molecular pathogenesis of the cerebral amyloidoses

GARETH W. ROBERTS, STEPHEN M.
GENTLEMAN and JEANETTE McKENZIE

Introduction

Dementia resulting from a neurodegenerative disease is a common phenomenon in the ageing population, with approximately 600 000 cases in the UK and 4 000 000 cases in the USA annually. As many as three-quarters of these cases may be accounted for by a single category of molecular neuropathology – a process of cerebral amyloidosis (Roberts, Leigh & Weinberger, 1993a).

Amyloidosis itself is a generic term describing the deposition of abnormal fibrillar proteins in extracellular and intracellular spaces. Regardless of their biochemical diversity, all types of amyloid proteins undergo conformational changes and assemble to form fibrils that are insoluble under physiological conditions.

Cerebral amyloidosis refers to a range of neurological disorders where the central feature of the pathological process is the altered or aberrant processing of a normal cellular protein, with its subsequent deposition as an insoluble amyloid deposit. This process lies at the heart of several neurodegenerative diseases that range from the commonplace, e.g. Alzheimer's disease, to the more exotic disorders such as prion disease. The diseases can be characterized diagnostically by the involvement of a particular protein whose metabolic misfortune lies at the core of the pathogenesis of the disease process.

This rationalization of the, often idiosyncratic, categorization of neurodegenerative disease has been made possible by recent advances in understanding the genetics, molecular biology and, ultimately, molecular neuropathology of various types of dementia. The purpose of this chapter is to present a didactic overview of the data that underlies the current classification of the cerebral amyloidoses.

Alzheimer's disease, Cortical Lewy Body disease, haemorrhage with cerebral angiopathy–Dutch type (HCHWA-D), haemorrhage with cerebral angiopathy–Icelandic type (HCHWA-I) and prion disease are all forms of cerebral amyloidosis. Each of these clinico-pathological conditions can be associated with a characteristic protein and thus classified according to its molecular neuropathology (Table 8.1).

Table 8.1. *Classification of human cerebral amyloidoses*

Disease	Syndrome	Characteristic protein
Alzheimer's disease	Dementia	β-Amyloid protein
Familial Alzheimer's disease	Dementia	β-Amyloid protein
Down's syndrome	Mental retardation/dementia	β-Amyloid protein
Sporadic cerebral amyloid angiopathy (CAA)	Cerebrovascular degeneration/stroke	β-Amyloid protein
Hereditary cerebral haemorrhage with amyloidosis Dutch type (HCHWA-D)	Cerebrovascular degeneration/stroke	β-Amyloid protein
Hereditary cerebral haemorrhage with amyloidosis Icelandic type (HCHWA-I)	Cerebrovascular disease/stroke	Cystatin C
Prion disease	Cerebellar/cortical degeneration	Prion protein

Between them the processes of cerebral amyloidosis involving different proteins give rise to a considerable variety of clinical syndromes, which has resulted in their historical classification as different diseases (for examples of clinical symptoms see Table 8.1). Despite this clinical variability there are a number of common features that help make the case for viewing the cerebral amyloidoses as a coherent class of neurodegenerative dementias (Table 8.2).

In this chapter we concentrate on Alzheimer's disease and prion disease. The two conditions have overlapping symptoms and the individual amyloid proteins involved are both encoded by cellular genes that are normally expressed in the

Table 8.2. *Common features of cerebral amyloidoses*

Gene coding for a precursor protein

Alterations in gene structure linked to amyloidoses

Constitutive cellular expression of precursor protein

Altered gene structure or physiological/environmental precipitant lead to enhanced systemic/focal expression or secretion

Mutant protein or enhanced protein levels partially resist or overload normal pathways of protein degradation

Breakdown fragments of the precursor proteins undergo conformational change and adopt a secondary β-pleated sheet structure

Conformationally altered fragments polymerize and form insoluble protease resistance fibrils

Fibrils coalesce to form amyloid deposits

Amyloid deposits can act as a stimulant to further pathological processes brain and other tissues. It is hoped that study of one may help illuminate the biology of the other.

Common features of amyloidogenesis

Although amyloidosis is heterogeneous with regard to the biochemical composition of amyloid fibrils and their anatomical distribution, there are common factors that may contribute to the pathogenesis of amyloid formation and deposition. These include (Table 8.2):

> The involvement of a precursor protein that encompasses an amyloidogenic amino acid sequence. In most cases, proteolytic low molecular mass fragments of the precursor adopt a β-pleated sheet secondary structure and polymerize to form insoluble fibrils resistant to further digestion. However, in other cases proteolysis of the precursor may not occur but rather the precursor proteins are susceptible to conformational changes which, in turn, lead to amyloid fibril formation.
>
> The elevation of serum or tissue levels of the amyloid precursor protein reflecting overproduction, impaired clearance or both.
>
> The abnormal processing of precursor proteins, which is probably the most complex issue in amyloidogenesis. In some cases, aberrant processing may be largely determined by the primary structure of the precursor itself, as has been proposed for genetic variants and certain sub-groups of immunoglobulin light chains. In other cases, incomplete degradation of the precursor has been attributed to an impaired cellular function.

β-Amyloid protein cerebral amyloidoses

This group of diseases includes both sporadic and familial Alzheimer's disease (AD), Down's syndrome, Cortical Lewy Body disease, and sporadic and inherited Dutch cerebral amyloid angiopathies (HCHWA-D). β-Amyloid protein (βAP) deposits are also present in vascular malformations and are the major components of brain amyloid in asymptomatic elderly patients.

These diseases have pathological accumulations of β-amyloid precursor protein (βAPP) amyloid fibrils as a common characteristic of their molecular neuropathology (Glenner & Wong 1984; Masters *et al.*, 1985; Figure 8.1). It is assumed that the process of β-amyloid accumulation is a core and early feature of the disease process.

The β-amyloid cerebral amyloidoses show a wide spectrum of clinical symptoms (see Table 8.1), the extremes being marked by the occurrence of sequential catastrophic haemorrhages in Dutch cerebral amyloid angiopathy (Van Duinen *et al.*, 1987) (where pathology is confined to the cerebral blood vessels) or the slow progressive cognitive decline found in Alzheimer's disease (where the pathology is primarily synaptic and neuritic). Given that Dutch-type

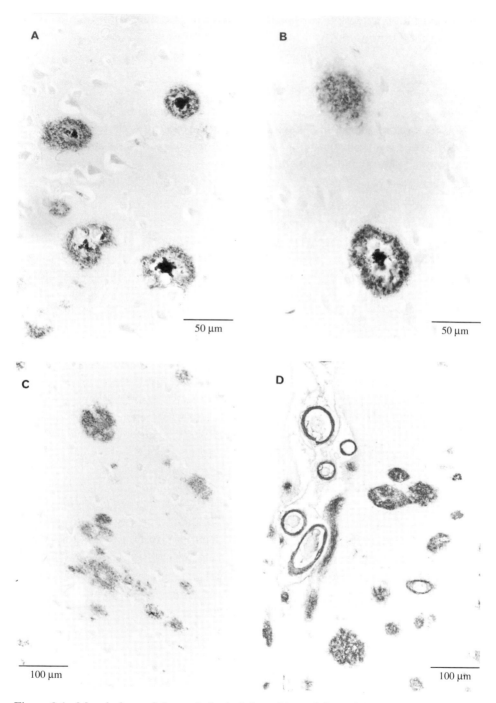

Figure 8.1. Morphology of the pathological deposition of β-amyloid protein. (A) Circular 'bulls eye' appearance of β-amyloid protein immunoreactive deposits within typical 'classic' plaques. (B) β-amyloid plaques show variable morphology, the two commonest forms being the diffuse and the 'classic' plaques. (C) The 'diffuse' type of β-amyloid plaque predominates in the early stages of the disease – example from a Down's patient

angiopathy is essentially familial and rare, and that the mode of amyloid deposition and plaque formation in Down's syndrome and Cortical Lewy Body disease is the same as in AD, we will concentrate on the pathophysiology of amyloid deposition in AD.

Causes of AD

The epidemiology of AD has been studied intensively. A number of putative factors have been implicated as being causal or associated with the pathogenesis of the disease. The best documented are increasing age, family history and a previous history of head injury (Roberts *et al.* 1993*a*).

Age

Increasing age has important effects on both the genetic and environmental precipitants of AD. In simple terms, an early age of onset is associated with a large genetic component (see below) but as the age of onset increases the effect of gene–environment interactions becomes more important. This is illustrated by the fact that Down's syndrome has the earliest age of onset (mid 20s) and appears to be a pure gene dosage effect (trisomy 21). Single gene-autosomal dominant forms of the disease (point mutations within the β-amyloid precursor gene) have an onset at 40–60 years of age, whereas polygenic disease involving several 'risk' genes has an onset between 50 and 70. Environmental events (e.g. head injury) interacting with genetic factors might be expected to have an onset between 60 and 80 years of age. Of course these are broad and almost certainly overlapping categories. However, the simplification serves to convey the spectrum from gene-dominated to environment-dominated initiation or triggering of AD.

Since the incidence rate for AD climbs dramatically with age (from $< 0.01\%$ below the age of 60 years to $> 25\%$ at 85 years and over) it seems reasonable to suppose that interactions between genes and environment underlie the majority of AD cases – a conclusion supported by the available epidemiology (Roberts *et al.*, 1993*a*).

Genetics

Approximately 20% of all AD cases are thought to have a predominantly genetic origin (Clark & Goate, 1993; Mullan & Crawford, 1993). From a wealth of studies over the past decade it has become clear that there are at

---

age 33. (D) All types of deposit 'diffuse' and 'classic' plaque and congophilic angiopathy can occur in the same brain regions.

least three distinct chromosome loci implicated in familial AD:

βAPP gene on chromosome 21
ApoE gene on chromosome 19
unknown gene on chromosome 14

Perhaps the most well-known are the mutations around the βAPP gene on chromosome 21 (Figure 8.2), including the substitutions reported at codon 717, close to the C-terminus of the βAP sequence (Chartier Harlin *et al.*, 1991*a*, *b*; Goate *et al*, 1991; Murrell *et al.*, 1991: Naruse *et al.*, 1991; Van Duijn *et al.*, 1991). Here, in a number of different families, a valine residue has been replaced by isoleucine, phenylalanine or glycine (Figure 8.3). Patients have been reported to have either typical AD pathology or a type of pathology that closely resembles that seen in Cortical Lewy Body disease. At codon 693, in the middle of the βAP sequence, a substitution of glutamine for glutamate has been observed. One amino acid away, at codon 692, an alanine to glycine substitution has been reported which gives rise to a variable phenotype of disease ranging from AD to HCHWA-D. More recently, a double mutation at residues 670 and 671 has been reported in a Swedish family (Mullan *et al.*, 1992).

Schellenberg and colleagues (1992) were the first to report a second gene, on chromosome 14, which was found to link with early-onset AD. As yet the precise identification of this gene is unknown but it has been localized to the middle of the long arm of chromosome 14. It is of interest that several genes in this area are known to influence the metabolism/processing of βAPP (e.g. α-1 antichymotrypsin, HSP 70). Although the identity of the gene remains unknown, it is thought to be responsible for the majority of hereditary early-onset AD cases.

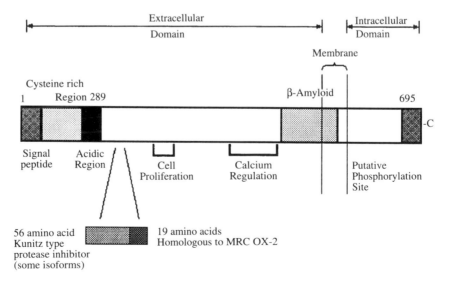

Figure 8.2. Structure of Alzheimer β-amyloid precursor protein.

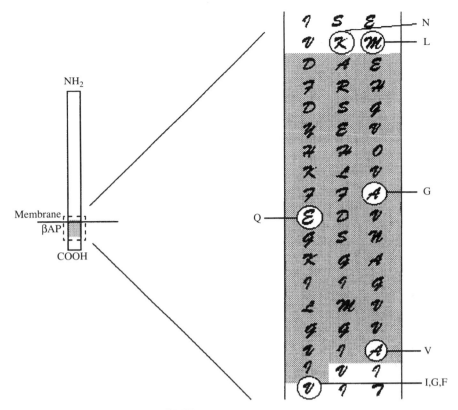

Figure 8.3. Mutation in the βAPP gene.

Until recently, genetic linkage studies have been restricted to early-onset AD cases but in 1993 Saunders, Strittmatter & Schmechel reported a genetic linkage for late-onset AD cases, on chromosome 19. The prime candidate gene in this region is the one for apolipoprotein E (ApoE), a protein involved in the transportation of cholesterol, which has been implicated in growth and repair during development or after injury.

The ApoE gene was already known as a risk locus for hypercholesterolaemia and coronary artery disease. Several tissues produce ApoE and it is most abundant in the liver and brain (macrophages and astrocytic glia). Although the role of ApoE in the liver is related to the control of plasma cholesterol, its function in other tissues is not fully understood. It is known that the four isoforms of ApoE (of which only e2, e3 and e4 are common) can have physiological effects of varying magnitude and direction. For example, e2 has a significant effect on lowering low-density lipoprotein levels in plasma whereas e4 can produce small increases. As a result the e2 allele is commonly regarded as atheroprotective and the e4 allele as atherogenic. The e4 allelle also shows an association with late-onset AD (Strittmatter *et al.*, 1993). Heterozygotes with the e4 allele are three times more likely to develop AD than people carrying the other ApoE isoforms. It has been proposed that the e4 protein has an enhanced affinity for the βAPP and as such may stabilize βAP fibrils – increasing the likelihood of βAP aggregation and deposition. In AD, ApoE has been found in extracellular senile plaques, intracellular neurofibrillary tangles and at sites of cerebral congophilic angiopathy (Namba *et al.*, 1991).

Head injury

There are a number of different lines of evidence for a link between head injury and Alzheimer's disease. A large number of epidemiological studies have been carried out, some of which show a significant correlation between head injury and AD, some that show a positive association and others that show no association at all. The variability of these results is due to the relatively small sample sizes used in the different studies. However, this problem has been overcome recently by the EURODEM consortium, who collected and pooled the data from the different smaller studies and performed a meta analysis (Mortimer *et al.*, 1991). This analysis confirmed that there is indeed a significant association between a history of head injury and the subsequent development of AD.

The other main body of evidence for a link comes from neuropathological observations. There are well-documented individual case reports in the literature where patients have suffered a single severe head injury and in subsequent years have developed a dementing illness (Clinton *et al.*, 1991). This phenomenon is also seen in boxers with dementia pugilistica or 'punch drunk syndrome'. In this case the repeated sub-acute trauma experienced in the boxing ring can result in a dementing illness very similar to AD some years after the boxer retires from the ring. It was confirmed recently that the pathology seen in the brains of dementia pugilistica patients bears all the hallmark lesions of AD, including large numbers of diffuse plaques (Roberts, Allsop & Bruton, 1990 and see Figure 8.1C for morphology).

The link between head injury and Alzheimer-type pathology was strengthened even further recently by the observation that serious head injury, resulting in death within two weeks, could initiate the deposition of diffuse βAP deposits within the brain (Roberts *et al.*, 1991, 1994).

βAPP structure and function

Since βAPP is considered to be central to these diseases, its gene structure, regulation and function require consideration (see Clark and Goate, 1993; Mullan and Crawford, 1993; Selkoe, 1993 for reviews).

βAP is a 39 to 42 amino acid fragment of a much larger precursor protein, βAPP (βAPP codons 672–714), which is a membrane spanning glycoprotein encoded by a gene located on chromosome 21 (Kang *et al.*, 1987; Dyrks *et al.*, 1988). Five different spliced transcripts of βAPP have been reported: βAPP 563, βAPP 695, βAPP 714, βAPP 751 and βAPP 770, with molecular weights ranging from 90 to 140 kDa, some of which contain a Kunitz protease inhibitor (KPI) domain (Figure 8.4).

The normally synthesized βAPP occurs either as a membrane-associated 110–130 kD species or a C-terminally truncated form, which is secreted from vesicles or released from the plasma membrane. In the nervous system, βAPP undergoes fast anterograde axonal transport (Koo *et al.*, 1990), and is thought to be active at the synapse (Breen, Bruce & Anderton, 1991; Schubert *et al.* 1991) where it interacts with molecules of the extracellular matrix.

Further clues as to the function of βAPP have come from studying the structural features of the various extracellular domains of the molecule. Based on such studies it has been proposed that βAPP is a cell surface receptor involved in the establishment and maintenance of cell–cell and cell–matrix

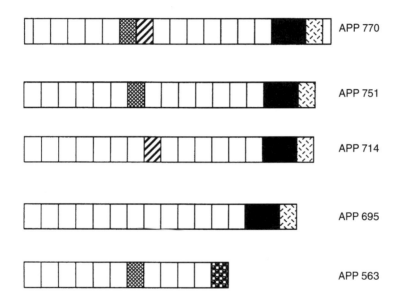

Figure 8.4. Alternative splicings of the βAPP gene.

interactions (Schubert *et al.*, 1991). The fact that the KPI-containing forms of βAPP (751/770, Figure 8.4) are identical with protease nexin II (Van Nostrand *et al.*, 1991) suggests that it may also have a role as a growth regulating factor (Oltersdorf *et al.*, 1989). The presence of the KPI isoforms in high concentrations in platelets also points to a potential role in the coagulation cascade and in wound repair and healing (Van Nostrand *et al.*, 1990).

A number of other, more speculative, functions have been proposed. βAPP has been described as a potential neuronal receptor mediating its effects via a G protein, G_0 (Nishimoto *et al.*, 1993). This proposal is based on the observations that βAPP binds to G_0 *in vitro* and that it contains a consensus amino acid sequence common to insulin-like growth factor, known to recognize and bind another G protein family member. This is intriguing but requires confirmation, since it is possible that the binding of G_0 may represent a step in the cellular trafficking of either βAPP or G_0.

The association with G_0 has also been raised in relation to the potential cytotoxicity of βAPP. G_0 is a calcium channel activator and it is thought that calcium influx might mediate some aspects of neuronal toxicity (see below).

Processing of βAPP

As mentioned previously, βAPP is present in several isoforms, produced by alternative splicing of a 19-exon gene on chromosome 21. βAPP 695 is the predominant form found in neuronal tissue while βAPP 751 is abundant elsewhere in the body. In each of these βAPP mRNAs, the 39–42 residue βAP is encoded as an internal peptide beginning 99 residues proximal to the carboxyl terminus of the βAPP and extending from the extracellular region (28 amino acid residues) into the putative membrane-spanning domain (11–14 amino acid residues) (see Mullan and Crawford, 1993; Selkoe, 1993, for reviews). It appears, therefore, that proteolytic cleavage of βAPP at both the amino and carboxyl ends of the βAP is necessary to generate the βAP found in amyloid deposits (Figure 8.5).

Considerable debate has ensued over the source of βAP and the site of the proteolysis of its precursor βAPP. The consensus is that the βAPP that forms amyloid plaques is of neuronal origin and is processed locally in the brain to form βAP, but multiple sites of origin (e.g. platelets, ependymal cells, choroid plexus) cannot be ruled out. In addition, further complexity could arise from the possibility that neurones in different brain areas or different classes of neurones within an area have slightly different patterns of processing.

Pathways to βAPP generation

A huge amount of experimental work has produced a reasonably consistent body of data indicating at least three main cleavage sites of βAPP. Further

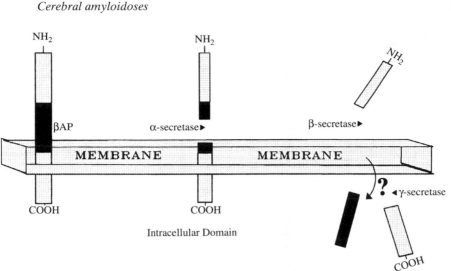

Figure 8.5. Alternative metabolic pathways for βAPP.

studies indicate that the fragment produced by these primary cleavage events can then enter three potential pathways for the processing of βAPP (Figure 8.5). The mechanics of the physiological relationship between these pathways is uncertain, although preliminary evidence suggests the existence of feedback loops that might bias processing from one route to another. These pathways have been inferred from the patterns of βAPP fragments that can be produced by cells. At present none of the enzymes that cleave at these sites has been identified. The three types of pathway are:

α-secretase pathway
β-secretase pathway
γ-secretase pathway

α-Secretase

This pathway is of considerable importance. The α-secretase site is in the middle of the βAPP sequence (residue 16 of βAPP and Lys 687 of βAPP) (Esch *et al.*, 1990; Anderson *et al.*, 1991). Thus cleavage of βAPP at the α-secretase site (just outside the transmembrane region) produces fragments with no amyloidogenic potential (Figure 8.5). The α-secretase activity produces a soluble N-terminal fragment and a membrane-bound 10 kDa C-terminal fragment (see Figure 8.5). This pathway is thought to cleave mature (*N*- plus *O*-glycosylated) βAPP during and after its transport from the Golgi to the cell surface. A membrane-associated secretase is assumed to be responsible for this process. However, the α-secretase seems to have no sequence specificity and appears to cleave the membrane-anchored βAPP at a set distance from the membrane surface (Sisodia, 1992).

β-Secretase

The second metabolic pathway for the breakdown has been characterized and is often referred to as a 'lysosomal/endosomal' pathway (Younkin, 1991). This enzyme cleaves externally to the membrane outside the βAP region and thus releases fragments containing intact βAP (Figure 8.5) (Estus *et al.*, 1992; Golde *et al.*, 1992). The actual site of this cleavage is not yet known but is thought to be at βAPP Lys670 or more probably Met671 (Hardy, 1992). This event produces the eventual N-terminus of βAPP (βAPP Asp672). Initially the α-secretase non-amyloidogenic cleavage was the 'normal' pathway for βAPP processing and the β-secretase activity producing βAP-containing fragments was a *de novo* pathological event. However, it has been shown that βAP is secreted normally from cultured cells (Haas *et al.*, 1992) and has also been detected in the cerebrospinal fluid.

The β-secretase cleavage is clearly a critical event in the pathogenesis of amyloidosis. At present the cellular localization of the cleavage event at Met671 is unknown. There was a considerable interest in the hypothesis that this could take place within lysosomes. However, the available data suggest that an acidic intracellular compartment other than the lysosome is involved. Although larger (11.4–11.5 kDa), potentially amyloidogenic, C-terminus fragments (containing the whole βAP sequence) appear in the endosomes and lysosomes, βAP has not been isolated from cell lysates, but only from cell media. Current evidence suggests that βAP may be produced in the Golgi or late endosomes.

Some of the β-secretase cleavage at Met671 probably occurs during secretory processing of βAPP at or near the cell surface. This is supported by the finding of a shorter secreted form of βAPP, apparently ending at Met671 in conditioned media. The cleavage at Met671 probably precedes the (γ-secretase) cleavage at Val711 during the generation of βAP. This is supported by the detection of a stable, 12 kDa carboxy-terminal fragment (beginning at/near Asp672) in βAPP-transfected cells. The quantity of this fragment increases in parallel with the increase in βAP generation in cells expressing a mutant form (βAPP 670/671) of the precursor.

γ-Secretase

The action of γ-secretase is to cleave βAPP within the transmembrane domain (at βAPP residues 711–714). The resulting fragments can then be secreted (Figure 8.5).

Following both α- and β-secretase cleavage of βAPP, portions of the resultant 10 and 12 kDa carboxy-terminal fragments undergo an additional cleavage in the region Val711–Thr714 (Figure 8.5). This creates the carboxy termini of the p3 and βAP peptides. The βAP peptide and a 3 kDa peptide (p3) also appear in the media of normal cells.

The p3 peptides are fragments of βAPP with sequences corresponding to the

C-terminus of βAP. Evidence suggests that the p3 fragments are derived from degradation of the N-terminus end of the 10 kDa membrane-bound residue of βAPP. It has been proposed that the production of p3 fragments may mark the flow of βAPP derivatives down the non-amyloidogenic endosomal–lysosomal pathway (Mullan & Crawford, 1993).

Effect of βAPP mutations on processing

In vitro studies using stable cell lines transfected with mutant βAPPs have provided useful evidence for assessing the effects of such mutations on processing of the precursor protein. The βAPP 670/671 ('Swedish') mutation results in a six- to eight-fold increase in βAP production accompanied by a decrease in p3 compared to non-transfected cells.

This type of information supports the idea that the pathways producing these two fragments are distinct but interdependent. The importance of this observation lies in the potential for disturbances in the regulation of these pathways to bias βAPP processing in the direction of βAPP production. Thus, ageing or AD factors that alter the regulation of these pathways (e.g. activation of protein kinase C increases production of C-terminal fragments) may contribute to the pathogenesis of amyloid formation.

Molecular mechanism of βAP fibrillization

βAP is a feature of normal cellular metabolism, is present in CSF and normal brains do not have an excess of amyloid deposition. On the basis of this it is clear that the mere presence of the soluble βAPP peptide does not lead inexorably to amyloid deposition. In support of this contention, a large number of studies have documented the observation that soluble βAPP peptides are non-toxic whereas fibrillar βAPP peptides can produce cytotoxic effects in cell culture. The processes governing βAPP fibrillization are critical for our understanding of the molecular neuropathology of AD.

The β- and γ-secretase cleavage sites produce amyloidogenic fragments that are considerably larger than the βAP 1–42 peptide. These potentially amyloidogenic fragments undergo further proteolysis to leave a heterogeneous series of βAP related peptides (including the major species βAP 1–39, 40, 40 and 42 and also βAPP peptides beginning at residues -6, -3, 4 and 11). The βAP peptides are able to aggregate into dimers and tetramers to form extracellular filaments (amyloid fibrils) 7–10 nm in diameter (Figure 8.6A).

To enable the process of polymerization to occur, the βAP peptides are thought to undergo conformational change and adopt a β-pleated structure. This appears to be a spontaneous event. At present the processes driving the conformational change are uncertain, as is the cellular site of the conformational change.

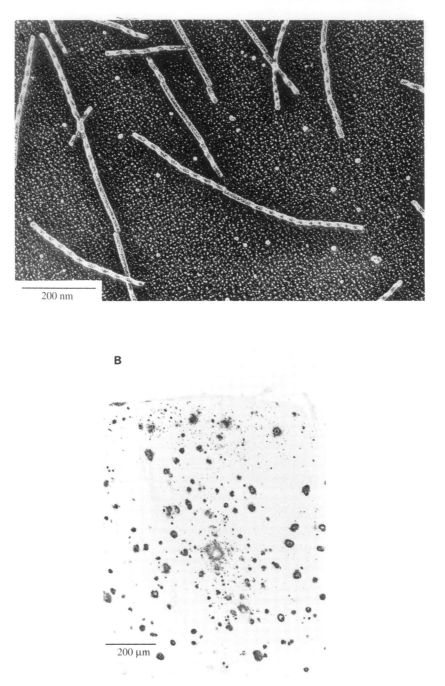

Figure 8.6. β-Amyloid 1–40 micrographs. (A) Transmission electron micrographs of synthetic β-amyloid 1–40 (Bachem ZK600) prepared by metal-mirror cryofixation followed by freeze-drying and rotary low-angle Pt/C metal replication. (K. H. Jennings, Analytical Sciences Department, SmithKline Beecham Pharmaceuticals.) (B) Extensive β-amyloid immunoreaction deposition is present throughout the cortex in Down's patients aged 50 years and over.

The results of a large amount of work to determine the critical parameters of βAPP polymerization and fibrillization can be summarized as follows (see Selkoe, 1993, for review):

βAPP residues 25–35 are essential
βAPP fibrillization is temperature- and pH-dependent
the length of βAPP peptides is critical
the concentration of the βAPP peptide is critical
the length of time in solution is critical

Deletion or substitution of βAPP residues 25–35 removes the ability to form fibrillar aggregates. Solubility of peptides up to βAP_{1-42} in size is dependent on pH and concentration. Peptides of up to 39 residues are largely soluble *in vitro* at pH 7.4, while βAP_{1-42} was significantly less soluble. Interestingly the βAP_{1-42} peptide is found in greater abundance in the cerebral plaques in AD while the βAP_{1-39} is the preferred species in cerebral vessels. Peptides longer than 42 residues were significantly more insoluble at pH 7.4. Aggregation is also dependent on peptide concentration and length of incubation in aqueous medium.

This data leads to the supposition that low levels of the βAPP peptide are less likely to fibrillize and are thus dealt with by normal metabolism – events that raise the focal concentrations of βAPP or alter local pH could lead to amyloid formation. These are points worth noting, since they underline the idea that relatively minor alterations in physiological parameters will allow the spontaneous aggregation of amyloidogenic proteins.

The conclusions drawn above are largely supported by *in vitro* observations on cell cultures expressing mutated βAPP proteins. The $\beta APP_{670/671}$ double mutation-derived amino acid substitutions are not integrated into the βAP peptide (the two codons encode the last two amino acids outside of the N-terminus, see Figure 8.3). Such changes are unlikely to result in longer and more insoluble βAP, rather they might cause an increase in the levels of normal length βAP 1–42. Recent work *in vitro* supports this contention by demonstrating excess βAP production in cells transfected with this mutation.

In contrast, C-terminus heterogeneity in βAP sequences (i.e. βAPP 1–39, 40, 41 and 42) in AD patients and the variable length of βAP products sequenced from transfected cells, suggest that the C-terminus is determined by carboxypeptidase action following the initial cleavage. The βAPP 717 mutation occurs at several amino acids after the C-terminus of the βAP fragment (Figure 8.3) and might be expected to interfere with this process, resulting in longer (more insoluble) βAPP fragments. However, increased length of secreted βAP has not been seen in transfected cell studies of the codon 717 mutations. Whether this phenomenon occurs in the human CNS is unknown. The issue might be resolved by sequencing the βAPPs in autopsy material from affected individuals in these rare codon 717, 670/671 families.

βAP cytotoxicity

AD is a neurodegenerative disease and fibrillar βAP seems to be cytotoxic in cell cultures. Studies of βAP neurotoxicity in culture indicate at least two broad concepts of mechanism to explain the cytotoxic effects.

One proposes that fibrillar βAP (Figure 8.6A) directly injures or kills cultured neurones, either by binding specifically or absorbing non-specifically to molecules on the cell surface. The other proposes that βAP generally causes little direct neurotoxicity by itself but can enhance the vulnerability of neurones to a variety of other common insults, such as excitotoxicity, hypoglycaemia or peroxidative damage. This lowering of the threshold for injury may be mediated in part by increases in intracellular free Ca^{2+} induced by βAP. Many further studies will be needed to establish the precise biochemical requirements for βAP to induce injury of neurones and to determine to what extent there exists a selective vulnerability to βAP among disparate classes of neurones. None the less, currently available data suggest that some βAP peptides can indeed exert trophic or toxic effects *in vitro* and that these are likely to be relevant to its biological activity in the brains of AD patients.

βAP and neurodegeneration

A simple hypothesis could be made to equate the neurodegeneration observed in AD with the presence of cytotoxic βAP deposits. It is clear from a consideration of the familial cases with βAP mutations and from patients with Down's syndrome (presumptive overexpression of βAP) that in these instances the overproduction or mismetabolism of βAPP is sufficient to trigger the full pathological spectrum of AD (Figure 8.6B). Unfortunately, things are not so simple. Whilst βAP deposits (plaques) are associated with degenerating neurites (see below) in many areas of the neocortex in AD, other areas such as the basal ganglia and the cerebellum contain βAP deposits yet show no obvious signs of degeneration. The interpretation of the observations in the human brain suggests that, whilst excess βAP production and subsequent fibrillization and deposition is a necessary pre-condition for the formation of plaques, other factors might also be required to generate the full spectrum of AD pathology.

This viewpoint is supported by the inconsistent results of the *in vitro* investigations that have sought to demonstrate βAP toxicity. Aggregation into fibrils is required for neurotoxic effects. However, such studies and pathological examination of human tissue suggest that additional factors are required to enhance the toxicity of βAP in the human CNS.

Examination of the brain of patients with Down's syndrome at different ages and of primates suggests this is the case. The full range of factors that might control either the ease or rate of βAP deposition and the subsequent evolution of neurodegeneration are still being identified. However, several factors of importance have already emerged. The role of ApoE as a genetic risk factor has already been discussed. ApoE proteins are also found within plaques and appear to be associated with the βAP fibrils. Complement proteins, heparan sulphate proteoglycans, microglia and astrocytes have also been associated with neuritic plaques. Clearly the formation of βAP deposits appears to be associated with, or more likely, triggers a complex cascade of molecular events that promote the degeneration of neuronal terminals and eventually cause the collapse of the cytoskeleton in neuronal cell bodies.

Pathogenesis of plaques and tangles

The exact sequence of these events is a matter of speculation at present (there being no suitable animal model or cell culture system in which to reconstruct these events). The full spectrum of brain amyloid lesions (including cerebrovascular amyloid, extracellular amyloid of senile plaques and intraneuronal amyloid of neurofibrillary tangles) is found in AD. Patients with trisomy 21 surviving beyond the age of 40 years develop the typical brain changes of AD (Figure 8.6B). Age-related analysis of the cortical lesions in Down's syndrome has shown that diffuse, pre-amyloid deposits immunoreactive with βAP antibodies may precede the appearance of plaques and neurofibrillary tangles. In addition the localization of βAPP in synaptic terminals (Schubert *et al.*, 1991) and the presence of increased βAPP immunoreactivity and βAP deposition in the vicinity of regenerating terminals in cases of head trauma (Gentleman *et al.*, 1993*b*) have led to the suggestion that βAP deposition occurs initially in the synaptic cleft (Gentleman, Graham & Roberts, 1993*a*; Figure 8.7). It follows from this idea that one of the earliest consequences of βAP deposition is some degree of deterioration or loss of synaptic connectivity. This loss of

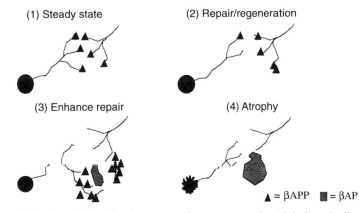

Figure 8.7. Potential role of regenerative processes in Alzheimer's disease. (1) βAPP is present in synaptic regions during normal neuronal activity. (2) Following damages, disconnection or other neuronal trauma, synaptogenesis is associated with increased local levels of βAPP. (3) Focal enhancement of βAPP expression can lead to βAP deposition (due to increased β-secretase activity) (Figure 8.5). (4) The resultant βAP deposit triggers the full blown AD pathological process.

connectivity could prompt further abortive regenerative activity (increased local production of βAPP) and thus initiate a pathological spiral leading to eventually neuronal destruction (Gentleman *et al.*, 1993*a*). This supports the idea that βAP deposition is an early event and might induce neuritic changes, rather than neuritic pathology occurring as a result of neuronal toxicity. This approach helps explain the observation of increased levels of βAPP expression and immunoreactivity following many kinds of CNS trauma (e.g. stroke, ischaemia, excitotoxic lesions) and has also been used to link the effects of age-related resprouting and the origin of Alzheimer-type pathology in the medial temporal lobe (Roberts *et al.*, 1993*b*).

The available data pieced together from neuropathological studies suggests the following sequence in plaque formation (Figure 8.8):

> **diffuse** – deposition of βAPP and slow aggregation into amyloid fibrils (involving binding to ApoE and HSPGs)
>
> **primitive** – involvement of degenerating/regenerating dystrophic neurites (involving activation of microglia, complement binding, tau phosphorylation, synaptic loss, disturbed Ca^{2+} metabolism)
>
> **classic** – condensation of amyloid core, development of spherical shape, degeneration of terminals and collapse of cytoskeleton to form tangles in neuronal cell bodies (tau phosphorylation, excitotoxic effects, astrocytic involvement)
>
> **burnt-out** – disappearance of degenerate terminals, relative absence of glial cells, condensation of amyloid into spherical core

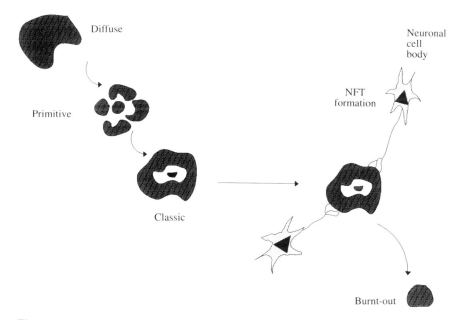

Figure 8.8. Possible evolution of plaque morphology.

This 'idealized' sequence of events lacks a formal scientific verification but allows us to conceptualize a long and complex pathological process. The sequence outlined above may take months or years to occur in the human brain. One of the problems in understanding the pathophysiology of the disease process has been in attempting to determine the nature of the events that might drive such a tortuous pathological process. Recent proposals have indicated that this type of pathology might be best conceptualized as a chronic inflammatory/acute phase response in the CNS and that in many respects AD could be analogous to an 'arthritis of the brain'.

Prion protein cerebral amyloidosis

A second group of disorders, now termed collectively as prion disease, also have an aberrant amyloid protein, the prion protein. This group of disorders encompasses scrapie and bovine spongiform encephalopathy in animals and Creutzfeldt–Jakob (CJD), kuru and Gerstmann–Sträussler–Scheinker (GSS) diseases in humans (Table 8.3; Prusiner, 1992).

Prion protein is a glycoprotein that is present in most organs and cell types, including neurones, and is expressed by these cells throughout life. Although its normal biological role is still unknown, the precursor has some structural similarity to a protein that modulates acetylcholine receptors, and may have essential 'housekeeping' functions, which may account for its high conservation between species. The gene encoding prion protein is located on the short arm of chromosome 20, and the longer of its two exons contains the entire transcribed 253 codon region of the gene. Data from a wide range of investigations have provided unequivocal evidence that PrP production is a normal event in a healthy brain. Therefore any pathological potential of PrP must result in an alteration in some aspect of its sequence, expression or properties. The only difference between normal prion protein (PrP^C) and pathological forms of PrP (PrP^{Sc}) found in the diseased brain is that PrP^{Sc} has increased protease resistance (Prusiner, 1991).

Table 8.3. *Prion disease*

Syndrome	Host
Creutzfeldt–Jakob disease (CJD)	Human
Gerstmann–Sträussler–Scheinker Syndrome (GSS)	Human
Kuru	Human
Scrapie	Sheep/Goat
Chronic wasting disease (CWD)	Mink/Deer/Elk
Transmissible mink encephalopathy (TME)	Mink
Bovine spongiform encephalopathy	Cattle

Genetics

Numerous point and insertion/deletion mutations have been reported in the prion gene (Figure 8.9). Of particular interest is a 144 base pair insertion (Owen *et al.*, 1989) at codon 53, where one affected family member developed CJD and another developed GSS. This finding implies that perhaps familial CJD and GSS form part of a spectrum of diseases in which prion protein plays a central role (Roberts *et al.*, 1993*a*). In fact, use of modern methods of gene testing has revealed different phenotypical representations of prion disease, e.g. fatal familial insomnia where a mutation was discovered at codon 178 of the prion protein gene.

Four PrP variants have been shown to be genetically linked to or track with inherited prion diseases. Substitution of leucine for proline at PrP codon 102 has been reported in three Caucasian and two Asian families. This substitution was not found in over 200 normal individuals. The codon 102 leucine variant is the only PrP mutation that has been formally linked to an inherited prion disease (Hsiao & Prusiner, 1990). Other mutations have been found to track with inherited prion diseases: a valine for alanine substitution at PrP codon 117 and a lysine for glutamate substitution at PrP codon 200 (Goldgaber *et al.*, 1989).

The possibility that the variant forms of PrP arise from alternative RNA splicing within the PrP gene can be eliminated as it is located within a single codon but alternative splicing of the protein itself or RNA editing are still possibilities (Figure 8.10).

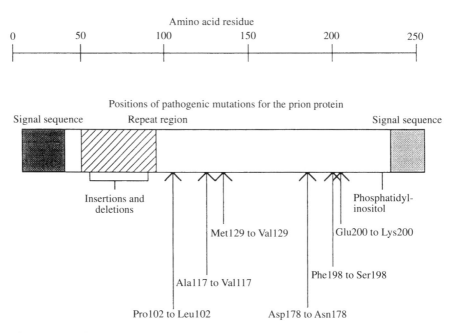

Figure 8.9. Disease-related disorders of prion gene structure.

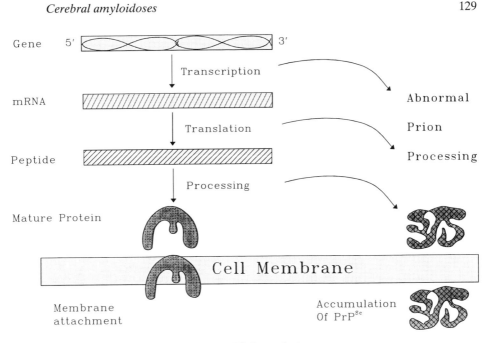

Figure 8.10 Possible pathway for PrP^{Sc} formulation.

The most likely explanation for the mechanism of conformational change is a direct protein–protein interaction. According to this hypothesis, the adherent isoform PrP^{Sc} comes into contact with the cellular isoform PrP^{C} and catalyses the conformational change from α-coils into β-pleated sheet (Figure 8.11; Prusiner, 1992). The site of conformational change is uncertain.

Metabolic labelling experiments with scrapie-infected cultured cells indicate that the conversion of normal to variant PrP is a post-translational event occurring either in the membrane or in the early stages of endosome formation (Caughey & Raymond, 1991). Structural studies indicate that both forms of prion protein are transported via the Golgi apparatus where their asparagine-linked oligosaccharides are modified and sialylated. Normal prion protein is presumably exported via secretory vesicles to the external cell surface where it is safely anchored (Stahl *et al.*, 1987, 1990). Variant prion protein, however, seems to accumulate within cells where it is deposited in cytoplasmic vesicles, many of which appear to be secondary lysozymes (McKinley *et al.*, 1991).

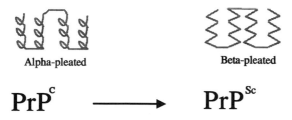

Figure 8.11. Prion protein alteration.

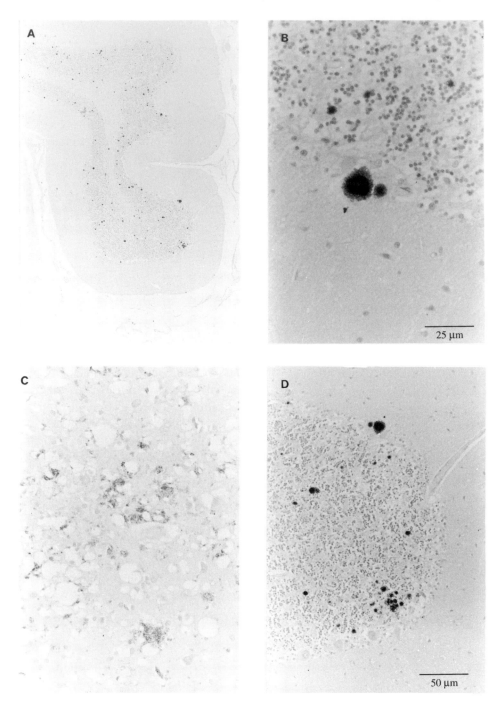

Figure 8.12. PrP^{Sc} amyloid deposits. (A) Low power of human cerebellum from a case of CJD. Note the large number of PrP^{Sc} immunoreactive deposits. (B) High power example of PrP^{Sc} plaque in human cerebellum. (C) PrP^{Sc} can also be found in 'diffuse' kinds of deposits in association with spongiform encephalopathy in the cortex in CJD. (D) PrP^{Sc} plaques can also appear as 'multicentric' in the human brain in Kuru and GSS.

The fact that variant prion protein is found in putative lysozymes within the cell may explain how it can enter cells. The conversion to the variant pathological prion state may occur on the cell surface (Figure 8.10). The cell then removes these variants from its surface by taking them up into secondary lysosomes. Normally these mutants would then be broken down and the constituent parts released back into the cytosol of the cell. However, the one property that distinguishes mutant prion protein is its resistance to proteolysis. Once it is taken up into the cell it disrupts the normal functioning of the lysosome and is released into the cytosol in its active form.

Based upon currently known molecular genetic information, the features of the inherited prion diseases that are determined by the primary structure of PrP appear to be: plaque formation and morphology, the topographic distribution of lesions, resulting in distinct clinical presentations and the host range (Figure 8.12).

The amyloid that is deposited in the CJD/scrapie model is providing further evidence that a neuronally-derived glycoprotein (PrP^{Sc}) can be changed into an amyloidogenic state that results in plaques and perivascular amyloid. The disease associations and mechanisms of amyloidogenesis of neuronal PrP is proving to be a most instructive model for AD.

Cystatin C cerebral amyloidosis

Cystatin C, also known as γ-CSF, γ-trace, or post-γ-globulin, is the third of the known cerebral amyloids and is the protein responsible for the Icelandic form of hereditary cerebral haemorrhage with amyloidosis (HCHWA-I) (Cohen *et al.*, 1983; Ghiso, Jensson & Frangione, 1986). Symptoms of HCHWA-I vary and may include paralysis and behavioural disorders as well as massive strokes that normally result in death before the age of 40. These clinical symptoms result from a build-up of cystatin C deposits, primarily in the cerebrovasculature (Butler and Flynn, 1961; Cejka and Fleischmann, 1973; Ghiso *et al.*, 1986; Benedikz *et al.*, 1989), although low concentrations are detected in other tissues (Gundmundsson *et al.*, 1972). It is a low molecular weight protein of 120 amino acid residues (Grubb & Löfberg, 1982; Abrahamson *et al.*, 1987) and a potent inhibitor of the cathepsins B, H and L (Barrett, Davies & Grubb, 1984).

Genetics

HCHWA-I is an autosomal dominant disorder arising from a point mutation in the cystatin C gene that causes a substitution of glutamine for leucine at residue 68 (Ghiso *et al.*, 1986). This mutation has been reported within affected members of eight HCHWA-I families (Palsdottir *et al.*, 1988) and is thought to lead to abnormal processing of the protein. The resultant amyloidogenic protein also lacks the first 10 amino acid residues.

The exact mechanism whereby the mutant cystatin C is deposited within the cerebral vasculature is unknown. CSF levels of cystatin C are higher than in serum (Löfberg & Grubb, 1979), and on the basis of the current evidence it would appear that the source of the protein within the CNS is most likely to be astrocytes, although both neurones and microglia also express low levels of the protein (Yasuhara *et al.*, 1993). In particular, immunocytochemical studies demonstrate marked staining in astrocytes around pial vessels and cortical microvasculature (Yasuhara *et al.*, 1993). Increased amounts of cystatin C immunoreactivity in pyramidal neurones have also been observed in patients with Alzheimer's disease but the significance of this to the molecular pathogenesis of the disease is unclear. This protein can also be found as a component of the vascular angiopathy in other diseases (usually in association with βAP) (Jensson, Thorsteinsson & Bots, 1986; Benedikz *et al.*, 1989; Maruyama *et al.*, 1990).

The resolution of the role of cystatin C in amyloidosis may have to await clarification of its normal function within the brain. It is known to be a secretory product of macrophages (Warfel *et al.*, 1987) and is thought to have a role in down-regulating or attenuating inflammatory processes (Leung-Tack *et al.*, 1990) and in the physiological control of regeneration (Sun, 1989).

Gelsolin cerebral amyloidosis

Finnish hereditary amyloidosis is an autosomal dominant disease (cf. Dutch- and Icelandic-type amyloidoses). The disease has been extensively studied in Finland (although a similar syndrome has been reported in the USA, the Netherlands and Denmark by, for example, Sack *et al.*, 1981). The disease may be related to a single founder and is thought to have originated in the 1400s (Meretoja, 1973). In heterozygous patients the disease onset is in the 20s and is characterized by progressive cranial neuropathy and lattice corneal dystrophy. In addition, there are systemic amyloid deposits. The amyloidogenic protein is derived from the actin-modulating protein gelsolin (Maury, Alli & Baumann, 1990*a*).

Genetics

A mutation in the gelsolin gene causing an amino acid change at position 187 (asparagine to aspartate) appears to be the cause in all patients suffering from the disorder (Maury *et al.*, 1990*b*).

Conclusions

Studies on the molecular genetics of cerebral amyloidosis have achieved two major objectives: the first is the unequivocal demonstration that aberrations in a given protein sequence cause these diseases, the second that these diseases can be classified on the basis of the molecular species which characterize their amyloid deposits. As a result, the study of the molecular neuropathology of cerebral amyloidosis has emerged as a new field of endeavour in neuroscience. The pathology resulting from aberrant protein processing and resultant amyloid fibril formation within the CNS is very variable. At present, attempts to equate particular symptoms or syndromes with specific gene defects have proved of limited value.

Despite the unitary concept of amyloid formation underlying these diseases, significant differences and similarities exist between them. The marked relationship between amyloid fibril formation and stroke in gelsolin and cystatin C amyloidoses is rarely observed in B and prion amyloidoses. The reasons for this are unknown but may relate to the length of the peptides which form amyloid fibrils. There are a number of similarities between the amyloidogenic processes underlying AD and prion disease. Both involve synaptic, transmembrane proteins. Studies of the accumulation of PrP and the formation of βAP protein from its precursor in AD suggest that the generation of the amyloidogenic fragments may occur in part in lysosome-related organelles (Mayer *et al.*, 1992). The release of hydrolytic enzymes from lysosomes may be a primary cause of neuronal damage in both diseases. Synaptic disorganization and loss is also a feature common to both diseases (Clinton *et al.*, 1993).

However, one notable difference between AD and prion disease is the lack of a local inflammatory process associated with the amyloid prion protein plaques in prion disease, which is seen in the βAP plaques (Eikelenboom *et al.*, 1991). This is demonstrated by the presence of microglial cells in and around βAP plaques expressing high levels of major histocompatibility complex (MHC) glycoproteins, immunoglobulin receptors, and complement receptors. Taken together with the appearance of other immune products it has been suggested that immune-mediated autodestructive processes may occur in AD (McGeer & Rogers, 1992; Royston, Rothwell & Roberts, 1992).

Neurone-to-neurone spread of the disease may occur in both prion disease and AD. It is thought that the spread occurs by a slow axonal transport (both anterograde and retrograde) and trans-synaptically. In AD it is not known what is transported but recent studies by Koo *et al.* (1990) have shown that βAPP undergoes axonal transport and Gentleman *et al.* (1993*b*) have shown that βAPP is found in damaged axonal neurones.

The molecular characterization of these diseases has opened the approach of designing transgenic animals bearing carefully engineered constructs. Such animals can be used to model aspects of the molecular pathology seen in patients and, more importantly, begin the task of devising and developing new therapeutic approaches to treatment.

References

Abrahamson, M., Grubb, A., Olafsson, I. & Lundwall, A. (1987). Molecular cloning and sequence analysis of cDNA coding for the precursor of the human cysteine proteinase inhibitor cystatin C. *FEBS Letters*, **216**, 229–33.

Anderson, J. P., Esch, F. S., Keim, P. S. *et al.* (1991). Exact cleavage site of Alzheimer amyloid precursor in neuronal PC-12 cells. *Neuroscience Letters*, **128**, 126–8.

Benedikz, E., Blöndal, H., Johannesson, G. & Gudmundsson, G. (1989). Dementia and non-hereditary cystatin C angiopathy. *Progress in Clinical Biological Research*, **317**, 517–22.

Breen, K. C., Bruce M. & Anderton, B. H. (1991). Beta amyloid precursor protein mediates neuronal cell–cell and cell–surface adhesion. *Journal of Neuroscience Research*, **28**, 90–110.

Caughey, B. & Raymond, C. J. (1991). The scrapie-associated form of PrP is made from a cell surface precursor that is both protease- and phopholipase sensitive. *Journal of Biological Chemistry*, **266**, 18217–23.

Cejka, K. & Fleischmann, L. E. (1973). Post-τ-globulin isolation and physicochemical characterization. *Archive of Biochemistry and Biophysics*, **157**, 168–76.

Chartier Harlin, M. C., Crawford, F., Hamandi, K. *et al.* (1991*a*). Screening for the beta-amyloid precursor protein mutation (APP717: Val–Ile) in extended pedigrees with early onset Alzheimer's disease. *Neuroscience Letters*, **129**, 134–5.

Chartier Harlin, M. C., Crawford, F., Houlde, H. *et al.* (1991*b*). Early-onset Alzheimer's disease caused by mutations at codon 717 of the beta-amyloid precursor protein gene. *Nature*, **353**, 844–6.

Clark, R. F., & Goate, A. M. (1993). Molecular genetics of Alzheimer's disease. *Archives of Neurology*, **50**, 1164–72.

Clinton, J., Ambler, M. W. & Roberts, G. W. (1991). Post-traumatic Alzheimer's disease, preponderance of a single plaque type. *Neuropathology and Applied Neurobiology*, **17**, 69–74.

Clinton, J., Forsyth, C., Royston, M. C. & Roberts, G. W. (1993). Synaptic degeneration is the primary neuropathological feature in prion disease: a preliminary study. *Neuroreport*, **4**, 65–8.

Cohen, D. H., Feiner, H., Jensson, O. & Frangionè, B. (1983). Amyloid fibril in hereditary cerebral hemorrhage with amyloidosis (HCHWA) is related to the gastroenteropancreatic neuroendocrine protein gamma trace. *Journal of Experimental Medicine*, **158**, 623–8.

Dyrks, T., Weidemann A., Multhaup, G. *et al.* (1988). Identification, transmembrane orientation and biogenesis of the amyloid A4 precursor of Alzheimer's disease. *EMBO Journal*, **7**, 949–57.

Eikelenboom, P., Rozemuller, J. M., Kraal, G. *et al.* (1991) Cerebral amyloid plaques in Alzheimer's disease but not in scapie-affected mice are closely associated with a local inflammatory process. *Virchows Archiv B. Cellular Pathology*, **60**, 329–36.

Esch, F. S., Keim, P. S., Beattie, E. C. *et al.* (1990). Cleavage of amyloid beta peptide during constitutive processing of its precursor. *Science*, **248**, 1122–4.

Estus, S., Golde, T. E., Kunishita, T. *et al.* (1992). Potentially amyloidogenic, carboxyl-terminal derivatives of the amyloid protein precursor. *Science*, **225**, 726–8.

Gentleman, S. M., Graham, D. I. & Roberts, G. W. (1993*a*). Molecular pathology of head trauma: altered βAPP metabolism and the aetiology of Alzheimer's disease. *Progress in Brain Research*, **96**, 237–45.

Gentleman, S. M., Nash, M. J., Sweeeting, C. J. *et al.* (1993*b*). b-Amyloid precursor protein (βAPP) as a marker for axonal injury after head injury. *Neuroscience Letters*, **160**, 139–44.

Ghiso, J., Jensson, O. & Frangione, B. (1986). Amyloid fibrils in hereditary cerebral hemorrhage with amyloidosis of Icelandic type is a variant of τ-trace basic protein (cystatin C). *Proceedings of the National Academy of Sciences, USA*, **83**, 2974–8.

Glenner, G. G. & Wong, C. S. (1984). Alzheimer's disease: initial report of the purification characterization of a novel cerebrovascular amyloid protein.

Biochemical and Biophysical Research Communication, **120**, 885–90.

Goate, A., Chartier-Harlin, M-C., Mullan, M. *et al.* (1991). Segregation of a missense mutation in the amyloid precursor protein gene with familial Alzheimer's disease. *Nature*, **349**, 704.

Golde, T. E., Estus, S., Younkin, L. H. *et al.* (1992). Processing of the amyloid protein precursor to potentially amyloidogenic derivatives. *Science*, **225**, 728–30.

Goldgaber, D., Goldfarb, L. G., Brown, P. *et al.* (1989). Mutations in familial Creutzfeldt–Jakob disease and Gerstmann–Straussler–Scheinker. *Experimental Neurology*, **106**, 204–6.

Grubb, A. & Löfberg, H. (1982). Human τ-trace, a basic microprotein: amino acid sequence and presence in the adenohypophysis. *Proceedings of the National Academy of Sciences, USA*, **79**, 3024–7.

Gundmundsson, G., Hallgrimmsson, J., Iondsson, T. A. & Bjarnasson, O. (1972). Hereditary cerebral haemorrhage with amyloidosis. *Brain*, **95**, 387–404.

Haas, C., Schlossmacher, M. G., Hung, A. Y. *et al.* (1992). Amyloid β-peptide is produced by cultured cells during normal metabolism. *Nature*, **359**, 322–5.

Hardy, J. (1992). Framing β-amyloid. *Nature*, **1**, 233–4.

Hsiao K. & Prusiner, S. B. (1990). Inherited human prion diseases. *Neurology*, **40**, 1820–7.

Jensson, O., Thorsteinsson, L. & Bots, G. T. A. M. (1986). Immunohistochemical comparison between the Dutch and the Icelandic form of hereditary central nervous system amyloid angiopathy. *Acta Neurologica Scandinavica*, **73**, 312–13.

Kang, J., Lemaire, H.-G., Unterbeck, A. *et al.* (1987). The precursor of Alzheimer's disease amyloid A4 protein resembles a cell-surface receptor. *Nature*, **325**, 733–6.

Koo, E. H., Sisodia, S. S., Archer, D. R. *et al.* (1990). Precursor of amyloid protein in Alzheimer's disease undergoes fast anterograde axonal transport. *Proceedings of the National Academy of Sciences, USA*, **87**, 1561–5.

Leung-Tack, J., Tavera, C., Gensac, M. C. *et al.* (1990). Modulation of phagocytosis-associated respiratory burst by human cystatin C: role of the N-terminal tetrapeptide Lys-Pro-Pro-Arg. *Experiment Cell Research*, **188**, 16–22.

Löfberg, H. & Grubb, A. O. (1979). Quantitation of τ-trace in human biological fluids: indication for production in the central nervous system. *Scandinavian Journal of Clinical and Laboratory Investigation*, **39**, 619–26.

Maruyama, K., Ikeda, S., Ishibara, T. *et al.* (1990). Immunohistochemical characterization of cerebrovascular amyloid in 46 autopsied cases using antibodies to β protein and cystatin C. *Stroke*, **71**, 397–403.

Masters, C. L., Simms, G., Weinman, N. A. *et al.* (1985). Amyloid plaque core protein in Alzheimer's disease and Down's syndrome. *Proceedings of the National Academy of Sciences, USA*, **82**, 4245–9.

Maury, C. P. J., Alli, K. & Baumann, M. (1990*a*). Finnish hereditary amyloidosis. Amino acid sequence homology between the amyloid fibril protein and human plasma gelsoline *FEBS Letters*, **260**, 927–32.

Maury, C. P. J., Kere, J., Tolvanen, R. & de la Chapelle, A. (1990*b*). Finnish hereditary amyloidosis is caused by a single nucleotide substitution in the gelsolin gene. *FEBS Letters*, **276**, 75–7.

Mayer, R. J., Landon, M., Laszlo, L. *et al.* (1992). Protein processing in lysosomes: the new therapeutic target in neurodegenerative disease. *Lancet*, **340**, 156–9.

McGeer, P. L. & Rogers, J. (1992). Anti-inflammatory agents as a therapeutic approach to Alzheimer's disease. *Neurology*, **42**, 447–9.

McKinley, M. P., Taraboulos, A., Kenaga, L. *et al.* (1991). Ultrastructural localization of scrapie prion proteins in cytoplasmic vesicles of infected cultured cells. *Laboratory Investigation*, **65**, 622–30.

Meretoja, J. (1973). Genetic aspects of familial amyloidosis with corneal latice dystrophy and cranial neuropathy. *Clinical Genetics*, **4**, 173–85.

Mortimer, J. A., Van Duijn, C. M., Chandra, V. *et al.* (1991). Head trauma as a risk factor for Alzheimer's disease: a collaborative re-analysis of case-control studies. *International Journal of Epidemiology*, **20** (Suppl.2), S28–S35.

Mullan, M. & Crawford, F. (1993). Genetic and molecular advances in Alzheimer's disease. *Trends in Neurosciences*, **16**, 398–403.

Mullan, M., Crawford, F., Axelman, K. *et al.* (1992). A pathogenic mutation for probable Alzheimer disease in the amyloid precursor protein gene at the N terminus of β-amyloid. *Nature Genetics*, **1**, 345–7.

Murrell, J., Farlow, M., Ghetti, B. & Benson, M. (1991). A mutation in the amyloid precursor protein associated with hereditary Alzheimer's disease. *Science*, **254**, 97–9.

Naruse, S., Igarashi, S., Kobayashi, H. *et al.* (1991). Mis-sense mutation Val→Ile in exon 17 of amyloid precursor protein gene in Japanese familial Alzheimer's disease. *Lancet*, **337**, 978–9.

Namba, Y., Tomonaga, M., Kawasaki, H. *et al.* (1991). Apolipoprotein E immunoreactivity in cerebral amyloid deposits and neurofibrillary tangles in Alzheimer's disease and kuru plaque amyloid in Creutzfeldt–Jakob disease. *Brain Research*, **541**, 163–6.

Nishimoto, I., Okamoto, T., Matsuura, Y. *et al.* (1993). Alzheimer amyloid protein precursor complexes with brain GTP-binding protein Go. *Nature*, **362**, 75–9.

Oltersdorf, T., Fritz, L. C., Schent, D. B. *et al.* (1989). The secreted form of the Alzheimer's amyloid precursor protein with the kunitz domain is protease nexin II. *Nature*, **341**, 144–7.

Owen, F., Poulter, M., Lofthouse, R. *et al.* (1989). Insertion in prion protein gene in familial Creutzfeldt–Jakob disease. *Lancet*, **1**, 51–52.

Palsdottir, A., Abrahamson, A., Thorsteinsson, L. *et al.* (1988). Mutation in Cystatin C gene causes hereditary brain haemorrhage. *Lancet*, 603–4.

Prusiner, S. B. (1991). Molecular biology of prion disease. *Science*, **252**, 1515–22.

Prusiner, S. B. (1992). Natural and experimental prion disease of humans and animals. *Current Opinions Neurobiology*, **2**, 638–47.

Roberts, G. W., Allsop, D. & Bruton, C. (1990). The occult aftermath of boxing. *Journal of Neurology, Neurosurgery and Psychiatry*, **53**, 373–8.

Roberts, G. W., Gentleman, S. M., Lynch, A. & Graham, D. I. (1991). βA4 amyloid protein deposition in brain after head trauma. *Lancet*, **338**, 1422–3.

Roberts, G. W., Gentleman, S. M., Lynch, A. *et al.* (1994). β-amyloid protein deposition in the brain after severe head injury: implications for the pathogenesis of Alzheimer's disease. *Journal of Neurology, Neurosurgery and Psychiatry*, **57**, 419–25.

Roberts, G. W., Leigh, P. N. & Weinberger, D. R. (1993a) In *Neuropsychiatric disorders*, Wolfe Publishers, London.

Roberts, G. W., Nash, M., Ince, P. G. *et al.* (1993b). On the origin of Alzheimer's disease: a hypothesis. *Neuroreport*, **4**, 7–9.

Royston, M. C., Rothwell, N. & Roberts, G. W. (1992). Alzheimer's disease: from pathology to potential treatment. *Trends in Pharmacological Sciences*, **13**, 131–3.

Sack, G. H., Dumars, K. W., Gummerson, K. S. *et al.* (1981). Three forms of dominant amyloid neuropathy. *Johns Hopkins Medical Journal*, **149**, 239–47.

Saunders, A. M., Strittmatter, W. J. & Schmechel, D. (1993). Association of apolipoprotein E allele E4 with late onset familial and sporadic Alzheimer's disease. *Neurology*, **43**, 1462–72.

Schellenberg, G., Bird, T., Wijsman, E. *et al.* (1992). Genetic linkage evidence for a familial Alzheimer disease locus on chromosome 14. *Science*, **258**, 668–71.

Schubert, N., Prior, R., Weidemann, A. *et al.* (1991). Localization of Alzheimer's βA4 amyloid precursor protein at central and peripheral synaptic sites. *Brain Research*, **563**, 184–94.

Selkoe, D. J. (1993). Physiological production of the β-amyloid protein and the mechanism of Alzheimer's disease. *Trends in Neuroscience*, **16**, 403–9.

Sisodia, S. S. (1992). Beta-amyloid precursor protein cleavage by a membrane-bound protease. *Proceeding of the National Academy of Sciences, USA*, **89**, 6075–9.

Stahl, N., Borchelt, D. R., Hsiao, K. & Prusiner, S. B. (1987). Scrapie prion protein contains a phosphatidylinositol glycolipid. *Cell*, **51**, 229–40.

Stahl, N., Borchelt, D. R. & Prusiner, S. B. (1990). Differential release of cellular and scrapie prion proteins from cellular membranes by phosphatidylinositol-specific phospholipase C. *Biochemistry*, **29**, 5405–12.

Strittmatter, W. J., Saunders, A. M., Schmechel, D. *et al.* (1993). Apolipoprotein E: high avidity binding to β-amyloid and increased frequency of type 4 allele in late-onset familial Alzheimer's disease. *Proceedings of the National Academy of Sciences, USA*, **90**, 1977–81.

Sun Q. (1989). Growth stimulation of 3T3 fibroblasts by cystatin. *Experimental Cell Research*, **180**, 150–60.

Van Duijn, C. M., Hendriks, L., Cruts, M. *et al.* (1991). Amyloid precursor protein gene mutation in early-onset Alzheimer's disease. *Lancet*, **337**, 978.

Van Duinen, S. G., Castano, E. M., Prelli, F. *et al.* (1987). Hereditary cerebral hemorrhage with amyloidosis in patients of Dutch origin is related to Alzheimer's disease. *Proceedings of the National Academy of Sciences, USA*, **84**, 5991–4.

Van Nostrand, W. E., Farrow, J. S., Wagner, S. L. *et al.* (1991). The predominant form of the amyloid β-protein precursor in human brain is protease nexin 2. *Proceedings of the National Academy of Sciences, USA*, **88**, 10302–6.

Van Nostrand, W. E., Schmaier, A. H., Farrow, J. S. & Cunningham, D. D. (1990). Protease nexin-II (amyloid beta-protein precursor): a platelet alpha-granule protein. *Science*, **248**, 745–8.

Warfel, A. H., Zucker-Franklin D., Frangione, B. & Ghiso, J. (1987). Constitutive secretion of cystatin C (γ-trace) by monocytes and macrophages and its downregulation after stimulation. *Journal of Experimental Medicine*, **166**, 1912–17.

Yasuhara, O., Hanai, K., Ohkubo, I. *et al.* (1993). Expression of cystatin C in rat, monkey and human brains. *Brain Research*, **628**, 85–92.

Younkin, S. G. (1991). Processing of the Alzheimer's disease βA4 amyloid protein precursor (APP). *Brain Pathology*, **1**, 253–62.

9

Intracerebral transplantation and functional recovery

HARRY F. BAKER and ROSALIND M. RIDLEY

It has been known for almost 100 years that fetal cortex transplanted into the brains of adult rats can survive whereas mature brain tissue does not. We know now that fetal brain tissue not only survives transplantation into adult hosts but frequently develops substantial fibre connections with the host. Recent investigations have concentrated on the ability of such transplants to restore function in previously lesioned or damaged brains. It is becoming clear that neural tissue transplantation is a valuable tool for neuroscientific investigation of brain function and leads to the hope that this technique might also form the basis of a new therapeutic approach to certain neurodegenerative conditions. There have been many different types of transplants within the central nervous system but we will concentrate on only two, involving the dopaminergic and cholinergic systems since these are particularly relevant to neurodegenerative disease.

Dopaminergic systems

Rat dopaminergic systems

The caudate nucleus and putamen receive major dopaminergic inputs from the substantia nigra and it is degeneration of these projections that leads to Parkinson's disease in humans. Bilateral injection of the neurotoxin 6-hydroxy-dopamine (6-OHDA) into the substantia nigra in rats produces a parkinsonian syndrome consisting of akinesia, aphagia, adipsia and general debility, although most of the experiments on dopaminergic tissue transplantations have made use of the asymmetrical behaviour that results from unilateral 6-OHDA lesions. Following such lesions the rats tend to rotate spontaneously towards the lesion side (i.e. ipsilaterally) and adopt an asymmetric posture. The animals also ignore stimuli presented to the contralateral side (known as contralateral neglect). When a unilaterally lesioned animal is administered amphetamine, the enhanced release of dopamine from the nigrostriatal projections on the intact side causes an increased tendency for the rat to rotate ipsilaterally. If, however, the direct dopamine receptor agonist apomorphine is administered, the rat rotates contralaterally, i.e. away from the lesion side, because the lack of dopamine input to the striatum on the lesion side has rendered supersensitive the post-synaptic dopamine receptor.

The first studies of the functional consequences of neural tissue transplantation were carried out using these unilateral 'models' of Parkinson's disease and involved the intracerebral grafting of small pieces of fetal ventral mesencephalic tegmentum containing dopamine cells. Björklund & Stenevi (1979) showed that following insertion of fetal dopaminergic tissue into a cavity, which had previously been prepared adjacent to and in contact with the head of the caudate-putamen on the lesion side, the amphetamine-induced ipsilateral rotation was reduced and, indeed, by 16 weeks post-transplantation the animal tended to rotate contralaterally. In addition, the reduction of drug-induced rotation was found to be correlated with the extent of dopaminergic outgrowth into caudate. Similarly, Perlow *et al.* (1979) showed that there was a reduction in apomorphine-induced contralateral rotation following intraventricular injection of fetal dopaminergic cells but not control sciatic nerve tissue. Both groups suggested that intracerebral transplantation of fetal dopaminergic cells could provide the basis for a treatment for Parkinson's disease. Indeed Perlow *et al.* (1979) went on to suggest that it might be worth looking at grafts of catecholamine-containing adrenal medulla chromaffin cells, which had earlier been shown to survive transplantation.

These early reports were followed by a series of experiments in which other aspects of 6-OHDA lesion-induced impairments were assessed following intracaudate grafting of fragments of fetal ventral mesencephalon. Using both unilaterally and bilaterally lesioned rats, no recovery was found in sensorimotor deficits; nor did the grafts prevent or overcome adipsia, aphagia or akinesia (Björklund *et al.*, 1980). The authors suggested that this reflected the failure of the grafts to reinnervate those parts of the striatum concerned with sensorimotor and consummatory behaviour.

Until then most transplantation experiments involved placing small solid pieces of tissue into prepared cavities resting on vascular beds or into ventricles in close proximity to basal ganglia. There had been reports of successful implantation of chunks of tissue into deep structures (e.g. by Das & Altman, 1971) but attempts to graft solid pieces of fetal mesencephalic tissue into caudate or diencephalon were generally disappointing with only few neurones surviving. Another, more successful, approach involved the stereotaxic injection of dissociated cell suspensions. Small pieces of fetal tissue are incubated with trypsin and, following removal of the enzyme by washing, the cells are dissociated mechanically by repeatedly sucking up and down a fire-polished pipette. Such cell suspensions remain viable for one or two hours and can be injected stereotaxically through a fine gauge needle (Schmidt, Björklund & Stenevi, 1981). Early experiments using this technique showed that dopaminergic cells injected into caudate, dorsal parietal cortex or lateral hypothalamus survived for at least several weeks and that those injected into caudate developed processes within caudate reminiscent of normal innervation (Schmidt et al., 1981). Further experiments showed that a variety of neurone types could be made to survive dissociation and transplantation, that there is a critical period in embryogenesis where cells taken for transplantation can survive, and that grafts of dissociated dopaminergic cells can overcome amphetamine-induced rotation in unilateral 6-OHDA-lesioned rats. Using cell suspensions, the relation between graft site and recovery of function can be studied more precisely than with larger solid grafts. For example, Dunnett et al. (1983) demonstrated that there was complete compensation of amphetamine-induced rotation in unilateral 6-OHDA-lesioned rats over the course of 3–6 weeks after injection of dopaminergic cells into dorsal caudate (compared with 2–3 months for solid tissue grafts). There was also some recovery of sensorimotor function following lateral striatal placement, but there was no functional recovery if grafts were placed in the substantia nigra or lateral hypothalamus.

Monkey dopaminergic systems

Most of the work in developing the techniques of neural tissue transplantation has been carried out in rats. There are a number of arguments, however, for extending these studies to primates. For example, the behavioural repertoire of monkeys may permit more detailed assessment of restitution of function than that of rats and, perhaps more importantly, more sensitive measures of deleterious effects may be obtained. Second, the optimum technique for transplantation may vary between species and it may be that the best methodology for clinical use in humans can only be worked out in primates. Third, it may be possible to measure more complex and cognitive functions in monkeys and this has proved to be the case when studying cholinergic tissue transplants, as will be described later. For obvious reasons, however, there have been far fewer intracerebral transplants in monkeys than in rats.

The first report of functional recovery following intracerebral transplantation in primates came in 1986 but these and subsequent studies by a collaborative team based in Yale and Rochester, USA, were described most fully by Taylor et al. (1990). These researchers employed the neurotoxin MPTP, which is known to cause parkinsonism in humans exposed to it as well as in a variety of non-human primates, although not in rodents. Even when administered peripherally, MPTP appears to act directly on the pigmented cells of the substantia nigra causing degeneration. A number of vervet monkeys (Cercopithecus aethiops) were injected with MPTP i.m. over a 5 day period and the development of parkinsonian features was assessed over a 3–4 week period. Small fragments of vervet fetal dopaminergic tissue were stereotaxically transplanted bilaterally into the caudate nucleus. Some of these animals showed substantial restitution of normal behaviour and a reduction in parkinsonian features (e.g. degree of bradykinesia). In addition, two animals that had been severely impaired and one animal that was moderately impaired were assessed on an object-retrieval task. These animals showed substantial improvements over time following transplantation. In contrast, those MPTP-treated monkeys transplanted with inappropriate control tissue showed no behavioural recovery and could not be tested on the object retrieval tasks. Biochemical analysis of the cerebrospinal fluid showed some recovery of dopamine metabolism in the animals with dopaminergic grafts, and brain immunostained with antibodies to tyrosine hydroxylase (a marker for dopamine cells) showed a small number of surviving dopaminergic cells, indicating that a pronounced behavioural recovery can be achieved with a modest increase in the level of dopaminergic activity in the caudate. However, the mechanism of the graft-mediated recovery is not understood as the following experiment demonstrates. Bankiewicz *et al.* (1990) reported the results of bilateral transplantation of fragments of dopamine-containing fetal ventral mesencephalon into the caudate nucleus in five rhesus monkeys previously treated unilaterally with MPTP (administered by injection into the carotid artery on one side). These animals were compared with other MPTP-treated animals receiving grafts of non-neural control tissue, or with prepared cavities only. There was good long-term survival of the fetal tissue grafts although there was no reinnervation of host tissue. However, behavioural recovery, though good, was no better than that produced by non-neural grafts or other control procedures. The authors suggested that the recovery of function may have been due to regenerative processes in the host, stimulated by the grafting procedure, leading to reinnervation of the host caudate by dopaminergic fibres that survived the MPTP treatment.

Other studies with MPTP-treated monkeys have employed the currently more usual technique of injection of donor tissue cell suspensions. For example, Freed *et al.* (1988) and Bakay *et al.* (1987) have examined a total of six macaques with bilateral MPTP-induced lesions and with bilateral or unilateral stereotaxic placement of fetal dopaminergic cell suspensions, either in caudate alone or in caudate plus putamen. Seven animals with lesions but without transplants were used for comparison. The four monkeys with best evidence of graft survival showed marked improvements in clinical ratings.

It is clear that large primates do not breed well enough in captivity to sustain a large programme of fetal tissue transplant research and a move to smaller New World primates is taking place. The common marmoset (*Callithrix jacchus*) is a very small monkey with a high and reliable reproductive rate and it is possible to produce donor tissue of a very precise gestational age. Both bilateral MPTP administration and unilateral 6-OHDA injections in this species have been used to produce models of Parkinson's disease. Fine *et al.* (1988) injected ten marmosets intraperitoneally with MPTP daily for 3 days and assessed them for the following 3 or 4 months. The animals developed profound bradykinesia, limb rigidity, postural abnormalities and diminished vocalization. Three to five months after lesioning, some monkeys were injected stereotaxically into putamen with either dopamine-rich fetal ventral mesencephalon cell suspension or dopamine-poor fetal striatal eminence cell suspension. Other monkeys were given solid grafts. Overall results suggested that these animals showed some locomotor recovery only after bilateral transplantation of dopamine-rich tissue. Histological analysis 5 months after transplantation of dopamine-rich cells revealed dense aggregations of cells immunostaining with antibodies to tyrosine hydroxylase with projections to the caudate. The degree of outgrowth was much better from the dissociated cell grafts than from solid grafts. Amongst other things, the experiment demonstrated that allografts of dopaminergic fetal neurones survived at 7 months without immunosuppression and that the grafts sent processes to those areas that normally receive dopaminergic innervation but not to those areas that do not.

The experiments discussed so far have concentrated on the effects of transplantation on general locomotor ability or drug-induced rotation in lesioned animals. More recently Annett and colleagues (1990 and unpublished) have been assessing the extent to which fine movement control can be restored in marmosets with unilateral 6-OHDA lesions. Graft-induced functional recovery is only demonstrable if the impairments produced by the lesions are reliable and long-lasting and since MPTP- and 6-OHDA-lesion effects can recover spontaneously, all the lesioned animals were screened for the required impairments. Any animal showing a substantial and spontaneous recovery of function was not included in the transplant phase. In addition, animals were assigned to a lesion-alone or lesion-plus-graft group on the basis of post-lesion, pre-graft scores on a number of behavioural measures so that the two groups were matched. Any improvements in the grafted animals, over and above that seen in the lesion-alone group, might then be ascribed to graft action. Injections of dopamine-rich fetal cell suspension into either caudate alone or caudate plus putamen produced markedly improved activity and decreased rotation in response to amphetamine or apomorphine, changes which were not seen in untransplanted animals or in those with tranplants into putamen alone. Investigations were also made of skilled movements. Overall there was no evidence that dopaminergic grafts produced recovery from the ipsilateral hand preference in taking pieces of food from a moving conveyor belt seen following unilateral lesion. However, there was some improvement in the animals' ability to retrieve food from within a tube although the time taken to complete the retrieval remained significantly longer than for control animals. Preliminary results (L. E. Annett, personal communication) suggest that unilaterally 6-OHDA-lesioned marmosets with grafts within the putamen show a reduction in contralateral neglect, not seen in lesioned monkeys with no grafts or with dopaminergic grafts within the caudate. The site of graft placement appears to determine the form of the behavioural recovery, suggesting that the graft is interacting with adjacent host tissue to alter function.

Work is now underway to define the optimum methods of transplantation, including the best age for the donor tissue. However, even while the methodology is being refined, early successes with experimental models have encouraged clinicians to apply these techniques to patients.

Human dopaminergic systems

Despite the relative paucity of data from primate transplant experiments, a large number of patients with Parkinson's disease have received intracerebral grafts, and, in fact, more humans than monkeys have now been grafted.

The first attempts to alleviate the symptoms of Parkinson's disease (PD) using autografts of adrenal medulla chromaffin cells were carried out in two severely ill Swedish patients (Backlund *et al.*, 1985). Tissue dissected from the patients' own adrenal glands was placed stereotaxically in the head of the caudate nucleus unilaterally under computed tomographic (CT) control. However, apart from some apparent slowing of the disease progression, there was no evidence of benefit, although there were no significant side-effects either. Two further, less severely affected Parkinson's disease patients were also transplanted with adrenal medulla tissue, this time in putamen, and again there was a transient improvement with no side-effects (Lindvall *et al.*, 1987). The first report of substantial improvements in PD patients following adrenal medulla cell autografts came from Mexico (Madrazo *et al.*, 1987). Adrenal tissue (totalling about 1 g in each case) was dissected into small pieces, which were placed unilaterally into freshly made cavities in the head of the caudate and in contact with cerebrospinal fluid. The first patient, a 35-year-old man, was seriously ill prior to grafting and, though showing some improvement on L-DOPA (L-dihyroxyphenylalanine), was unable to tolerate the drug. He was more affected on the right-hand side, was rigid, bradykinetic, and had a resting tremor. By 17 days after transplantation he was able to walk; by 5 months he could walk without assistance, speak clearly and did not require drugs; by 10 months he could play football with his child and could visit the out-patient department unaided. The second patient, who was younger than the first, showed similar improvements after grafting. Since these early, dramatic improvements were reported and despite the earlier, less encouraging reports by the Swedish group, many Parkinson's disease patients around the world have undergone adrenal medulla autografting. However, evidence of a beneficial effect has not been well documented and there is an associated risk of morbidity and mortality. In the summary report of 106 Hispanic patients with adrenal medulla autografts, nine had died and a number had experienced complications such as respiratory problems, hallucinations and urinary tract infections (Madrazo *et al.*, 1989). In a recent review of the transplantation of adrenal tissue into the central nervous system, Fine (1990) calculated that, of the patients discussed at the United Parkinson's Foundation third workshop on adrenal transplants in Parkinson's disease (held in November, 1988), about 20% showed transient or persistent improvements in motor performance. Fine also pointed out that older, more severely ill patients were less likely to benefit from transplantation or were more likely to suffer morbidity. In those transplanted patients who have subsequently died, post-mortem examinations have generally revealed no surviving transplanted cells. This has been the case even for those patients who have shown symptomatic improvements during several months post-transplantation (Lieberman *et al.*, 1990). In addition, Garcia-Flores *et al.* (1990) performed MRI scans on nine patients between 3 and 12 months after transplantation of adrenal medulla grafts. In all cases they found cystic cavities at the site of transplantation within the basal ganglia and concluded that transplanted tissue had not survived, again raising the question of how these transplants exert such beneficial effects as they do. We will return to this matter later.

The first reports of the transplantation of human fetal dopaminergic cells into the basal ganglia of Parkinson's disease patients also came from the Mexican group (Madrazo *et al.*, 1988). Two patients were grafted; one was given fetal ventral mesencephalic tissue and the other was given fetal adrenal medulla tissue. The tissue was derived from a spontaneous abortion at 13 weeks in a woman with a history of cervico-uterine incompetence. Madrazo *et al.* (1988) suggested that since this procedure required the recipient to undergo only one rather than the two operations needed for autotransplantation, it would be associated with lower morbidity, especially in the more elderly patients. However, the grafted tissue is not host derived and some surgeons have addressed the possibility of tissue rejection by maintaining patients on immune suppressant drugs such as cyclosporine and steroids. The first two patients to receive fetal tissue grafts were reported 8 weeks later to have shown evident objective improvement in the symptoms of Parkinson's disease (Madrazo *et al.*, 1988). As with autografting of adrenal medulla tissue, however, transplantation of fetal dopaminergic cells in Parkinson's disease patients has not fulfilled the expectations generated by the early reports. The first two Swedish patients to receive fetal dopamine-rich mesencephalic tissue grafts did not improve during a 6 month post-operative observation period, prompting the authors to conclude that 'neural transplantation is still an experimental approach, and not a therapeutic alternative in Parkinson's disease' (Lindvall *et al.*, 1989). They went on to stress the importance of developing the methodology in animal studies in parallel with assessing grafting procedures in patients. But again, as with the adrenal medulla autografts, the variable outcome of the early fetal mesencephalic tissue transplants has not deterred neurosurgeons from carrying out quite a large number of these transplants in various centres thought the world, including more than 30 in Britain. The techniques have varied somewhat, e.g. between an open surgical approach and a stereotaxic delivery; donor tissue between 6 and 19 weeks gestational age; in caudate and/or putamen target sites; immunosuppression and no immunosuppression. It is too early to say with any confidence whether or not fetal neural tissue transplantation will be of long-term therapeutic benefit in Parkinson's disease since few longitudinal studies have been carried out. Several groups (e.g.

Hitchcock *et al.*, 1990; Lindvall *et al.*, 1990) have concluded, however, that there often is a definite improvement after transplantation and it does appear that fetal neural tissue grafts can show good long-term survival. Why there should be considerable variability between the results reported by different groups is not known but is likely to reflect the different surgical techniques and the rigour of behavioural measurement.

Lindvall & Björklund (1989) have stressed the importance of quantitative assessment of the patient's symptoms and the progression of the illness before transplantation. They point out that this aspect has varied between different studies and has made comparison difficult. They also draw attention to the relatively few attempts to establish whether dopamine neurones survive and reinnervate host tissue. Lindvall *et al.* (1990) have addressed these points in their recent clinical reports. One patient, a 49-year-old man, was assessed thoroughly for 11 months prior to transplantation. Although he had been treated successfully with L-DOPA he was developing worsening 'on–off' phenomena. During 'off' phases, comprising 40–50% of the time, he was rigid and hypokinetic with a right arm tremor. He was given a 6-L-[^{18}F]-fluorodopa positron emission tomographic (PET) scan 12 months before surgery, which established that the left putamen was low in dopamine synthesizing capacity. Pooled dissociated mesencephalic tissue from four fetuses (aged 8–9 weeks) was implanted stereotaxically into the left putamen. The patient's progress over a 5 month post-operative period was monitored. Two to 3 months after transplant there was a sharp reduction in the amount and frequency of 'off' periods, which was sustained. There was also a reduction in the time taken to execute simple movements. Another PET scan at 5 months after transplantation showed a substantial improvement in dopamine-synthesizing capacity in the left putamen. It should be pointed out that this patient was maintained on a constant drug regime throughout the entire study period. This obviates the problem of variation in clinical picture in response to variation in drug regime. The long pre-operative assessment period allowed the investigators to establish that the symptomatology was very stable over a period of 11 months.

It has been thought by some that the improvement in symptoms following transplantation could result from damage to the blood–brain barrier, allowing easier access of L-DOPA to the brain. However, as Lindvall *et al.* (1990) pointed out, the grafted neuronal tissue establishes a well-developed blood–brain barrier within 1 to 2 weeks of implantation and their patient showed no symptomatic improvement during that immediate post-operative period. Indeed, these authors went on to report that the procedural modifications they used in this patient, which include a small-diameter delivery instrument and better handling of the tissue, led to less tissue damage at the graft site and better survival of dopamine neurones. Despite the encouraging results in this patient (and more recent reports suggest that his improved performance persists), Lindvall and colleagues remain cautious in their advocacy of fetal neural transplantation as an effective therapy for Parkinson's disease and reiterate their earlier argument that methodology must be developed further (Lindvall *et al.*, 1990).

Cholinergic systems

Rat cholinergic systems

Studies on the ability of transplants of cholinergic-rich fetal neural tissue to overcome the effects of lesions of the cholinergic system have been carried out in parallel with work on the dopaminergic system. The emphasis, however, is different. Whereas the dopaminergic transplant field has concerned itself with movement disorders and relates, ultimately, to the symptoms and impairments seen in Parkinson's disease, cholinergic transplants address the issues of cognition, learning and memory. The impetus for this emphasis derives from the finding that a major neurochemical deficit found in Alzheimer's disease and other neurodegenerative diseases that are accompanied by marked cognitive impairment, is a profound loss of cholinergic innervation of cortical and limbic areas. Post-mortem analysis of the brains of those dying with Alzheimer's disease demonstrates a marked reduction in the activity of choline acetyltransferase (ChAT) in neocortex, hippocampus and entorhinal cortex (Bowen *et al.*, 1976; Davies & Maloney, 1976; Perry *et al.*, 1977; Rossor *et al.*, 1984). The cells of origin of the major cholinergic systems lie within the basal forebrain in the basal nucleus of Meynert (with projections to cortex and amygdala) and the vertical limb of the diagonal bond of Broca (with projections to hippocampus and entorhinal cortex). There is considerable evidence of loss of these cholinergic cells in the brains of Alzheimer patients (Nakano & Hirano, 1982; Whitehouse *et al.*, 1982), and a contribution of this cholinergic dysfunction to the cognitive symptoms of dementia is indicated by the correlation between low mental test score in life and loss of ChAT activity measured post-mortem (Perry *et al.*, 1978, 1985). Since the original findings of cholinergic losses were reported, a number of other biochemical and morphological changes have been described that may contribute to the cognitive impairments in Alzheimer's disease (Bondareff, Mountjoy & Roth, 1981; Cross *et al.*, 1981; Roberts, Crow & Polak, 1985). However, and despite the views held by some (e.g. Fibiger, 1991), it is still widely accepted that the cholinergic losses found in Alzheimer's disease are in large part responsible for the cognitive decline that is such a key feature of the disease.

The major cholinergic projection from the septum and diagonal band to the hippocampus runs through the fornix. Early experiments by Bjorklund & Stenevi (1977) demonstrated that embryonic septal neurones transplanted into the hippocampus of adult rats with lesions of the fornix could survive and form anatomically specific patterns of cholinergic connectivity that resembled normal innervation. The first studies of the ability of cholinergic grafts to restore learning ability in rats with lesions of the fornix were published in 1982

(Dunnett *et al.*, 1982; Low *et al.*, 1982). Transection of the fornix cuts not only the cholinergic projections to the hippocampus but also noradrenergic and other subcortical connections as well. Dunnett *et al.* (1982) assessed the ability of fetal septal and fetal locus coeruleus tissue grafts into hippocampus in fornix-transected rats to restore the rats' ability to learn an alternation procedure in a T-maze. Only fetal cholinergic-rich septal grafts were behaviourally beneficial and the degree of recovery was significantly correlated with the degree of AChE-positive fibre in-growth into the hippocampus. Low *et al.* (1982) used an eight-arm radial maze to assess the capacity of fetal septal tissue transplants to overcome the learning impairments produced by fornix-transection. In this case, however, there was no obvious improvement in learning unless the animals were treated, prior to testing, with the acetylcholinesterase inhibitor, physostigmine.

Since these early experiments were published a number of other tasks have been used to tax the learning ability of fornix-transected rats and evaluate the ameliorating effects of fetal neural tissue transplants. This work has been reviewed extensively by Dunnett (1990). By and large, functional recovery in fornix-transected rats has been less than complete and this may reflect the fact that the fornix carries other, non-cholinergic hippocampal efferents and afferents. Rather better functional recovery has been seen in aged rats receiving intrahippocampal fetal septal grafts. Aged rats, screened for impaired performance in a Morris water-maze, were reassessed 3 months after grafting. When compared to non-grafted control animals who remained impaired on water-maze performance, the grafted animals were much improved and in some animals performance was as good as that seen in control, non-impaired animals (Gage *et al.* 1984). Arendt *et al.* (1988) have made use of a different model of amnesia to assess the efficacy of fetal cholinergic tissue transplants. Alcohol-induced Korsakoff's syndrome in humans is characterized by a variety of neuropathological changes including marked losses in central cholinergic and noradrenergic markers, which are accompanied by severe and apparently irreversible memory deficits. Arendt and colleagues showed that rats that were administered high levels of alcohol in their drinking water over a 6-month period followed by a 1-month washout period were markedly impaired at learning both working (short-term) and reference (long-term) memory tasks in an eight-arm radial maze. A reassessment of learning ability in these rats was started 14 days after transplantation of fetal cholinergic-rich tissue into hippocampus, cortex, or hippocampus plus cortex. There was a general overall improvement in learning ability over the following 9 weeks, especially in those rats receiving transplants into both cortex and hippocampus. In a similar experiment, Hodges *et al.* (1990) looked at the effects of cholinergic-rich (septal) and cholinergic-poor (hippocampal) fetal grafts on the performance of neurotoxin-lesioned rats in an eight-arm radial maze. Rats were lesioned by ibotenic acid injections into nucleus basalis, medial septum and diagonal band, which destroy cholinergic inputs into hippocampus, amygdala and cortex.

These animals were impaired on both working and reference memory components. As in the earlier experiment by Arendt *et al.* (1988) cholinergic-rich
grafts within cortex, hippocampus or both produced an improvement in the
animals' performance on this task. Rats receiving cholinergic-rich transplants
into the basal forebrain showed no evidence of functional recovery, and
lesioned animals receiving no grafts or cholinergic-poor grafts performed
significantly worse than controls throughout.

Monkey cholinergic systems

The common marmoset (*Callithrix jacchus*) is the only primate that has been
used for assessing the effects of cholinergic transplants on cognitive function.
For some time we have been studying the cognitive effects of both neurotoxic
and surgical lesions of the cholinergic projections in this species and have
established that the resulting cognitive impairments are essentially the same as
those seen following the surgical removal of target areas. We have also
demonstrated that the cognitive deficits produced by cholinergic lesions can be
ameliorated by direct administration of cholinergic agonists such as pilocarpine
and arecoline (Ridley *et al.*, 1986, 1988, 1991). The results of these experiments provide evidence that normal cognitive function does not depend
specifically on patterned information carried within the cholinergic projection
but, rather, that these projections have a modulatory or enabling effect on
cortical or hippocampal function, analogous to the enabling role of ascending
dopamine projections in motor systems (Ridley *et al.*, 1986). In our cholinergic
transplantation studies we have concentrated on the projections from the
diagonal band through the fornix to the hippocampus. Monkeys with bilateral
transection of the fornix are severely, but selectively, impaired at learning
visuospatial conditional tasks (Ridley *et al.*, 1991). This impairment is quite
specific; fornix-transected monkeys are able to learn tasks in which they have
to choose one of two different objects presented simultaneously (i.e. a two-
choice, visual object discrimination task). This pattern of impairment in
monkeys is the same as that seen following selective hippocampal dysfunction
(Ridley & Baker, 1991), whereas impaired performance on the visual-object
discrimination task usually occurs as a consequence of damage to surrounding
cortex.

After assessing the degree of impairment we transplanted cholinergic-rich
cell suspensions prepared from marmoset fetuses bilaterally into the hippocampus of a number of these lesioned monkeys. As a control procedure, a further
group of lesioned monkeys was transplanted with non-cholinergic, fetal hippocampal tissue. Three months after transplantation, the grafted animals,
together with a group of lesioned, non-transplanted animals were tested on a
wide range of learning tasks. While the fornix-transected, non-grafted animals
remained impaired on visuospatial tasks throughout the lengthy test period, the

performance of the lesioned animals with cholinergic grafts had recovered and was undistinguishable from that of control animals. On the other hand, the lesioned animals with non-cholinergic grafts showed no improvement on visuospatial tasks. At the end of testing, the brains of all the animals were examined by acetylcholinesterase histochemistry. Densely staining grafts were seen bilaterally within the temporal lobes of animals with cholinergic grafts, with substantial fibre outgrowth into surrounding host tissue (Ridley *et al.*, 1991). This experiment was the first to demonstrate that cholinergic-rich grafts can restore cognitive abilities in primates with lesions within the cholinergic system (See Figures 9.1–9.3).

As is the case for the dopaminergic grafts discussed earlier, there are a number of mechanisms by which grafts may induce recovery in the host and these have been reviewed by Björklund and colleagues (1987). For example, grafts could exert their effects through a general, diffuse release of hormones or neurotransmitters, although in the marmoset experiment just cited this is an unlikely explanation because acetylcholine is broken down too quickly to act at a distance from the point of release. Or they may stimulate regeneration within

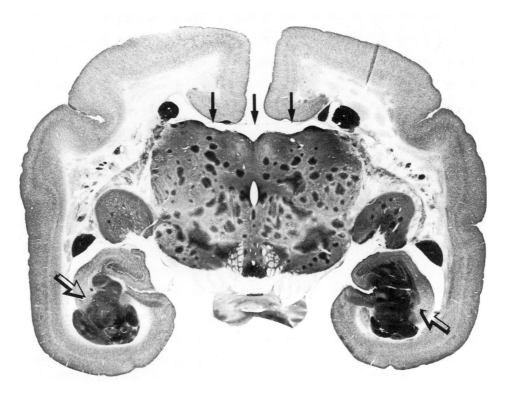

Figure 9.1. Coronal section of marmoset brain stained for acetylcholinesterase. Filled arrows indicate bilateral ablation of fornix and overlying corpus callosum. Open arrows indicate grafts of fetal cholinergic-rich neural tissue into the temporal lobes.

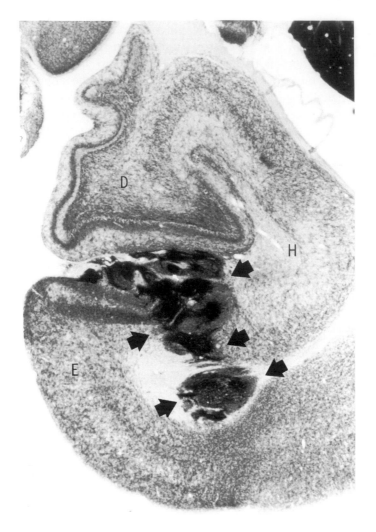

Figure 9.2. Temporal lobe of marmoset brain stained for acetylcholinesterase. Arrows indicate graft of fetal cholinergic-rich neural tissue. Cholinesterase staining (which is diminished by fornix transection) is restored by graft in dentate gyrus (D), hippocampus (H) and entorhinal cortex (E).

host tissue by supplying trophic factors, although in the marmoset experiment such trophic factors would have to be specific to each type of transplanted tissue, because grafts of cholinergic-rich septal tissue produced behavioural recovery and near-normal patterns of acetylcholinesterase staining, while cho-linergic-poor hippocampal grafts did not. Finally, grafts may make functional connections with host tissue and there is ultrastructural evidence to suggest that they do so (Clarke *et al.*, 1986, 1990). Neurophysiological experiments also show that septal tissue grafts restore acetylcholine release in the host hippo-campus and that this release is under host control (Nilsson *et al.*, 1990).

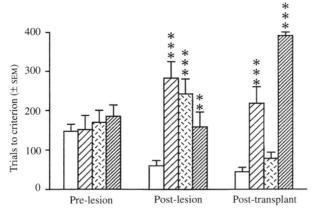

Figure 9.3. This histogram shows the effect on learning ability of fornix transection and subsequent transplantation of cholinergic-rich or cholinergic-poor neural tissue into the hippocampus of marmosets. Four groups of marmosets were first taught a visuospatial conditional task to a predetermined criterion. In this task they had to learn to choose the stimulus on the left if one pair of identical objects was presented and the stimulus on the right if another pair of identical objects was presented. Three groups then received bilateral transection of the fornix, which cuts off the cholinergic projection to the hippocampus. These three groups were impaired at learning another visuospatial conditional task. Three months after transplantation of fetal cholinergic-rich neural tissue into the hippocampus of fornix-lesioned animals, marmosets were no longer impaired at learning this type of task whereas fornix-lesioned animals with no transplant or with transplants of fetal cholinergic-poor neural tissue into the hippocampus remained severely impaired. □ Control monkeys, $n = 12$. ▨ Monkeys with fornix transection only, $n = 10$. ▦ Monkeys with fornix transection and transplants of cholinergic-rich neural tissue, $n = 8$. ▨ Monkeys with fornix transection and transplants of cholinergic-poor neural tissue, $n = 4$. Pre-lesion the groups did not differ in their learning ability. Post-lesion all three groups with fornix transection were impaired relative to control groups. Post-transplant the fornix-only groups and group transplanted with cholinergic-poor tissue remained severely impaired, but the group with fornix transection and transplants of cholinergic-rich tissue were completely restored in their learning ability. $**p < 0.01$; $***p < 0.001$.

Human cholinergic systems

As we have seen, the replacement of a single neurotransmitter deficit (dopamine) in Parkinson's disease by fetal neural tissue transplantation is now being studied extensively. However, although degeneration of the cholinergic projection systems is a feature of a number of neurodegenerative conditions including Alzheimer's disease (Bowen *et al.*, 1976), Parkinson's disease with dementia (Perry *et al.*, 1985) and Korsakoff's syndrome (Arendt *et al.*, 1983), the widespread and often severe pathology in the target areas of these projection systems may markedly reduce the potential efficacy of cholinergic transplants in these diseases. On the other hand, since cholinergic loss does lead to cognitive impairment in humans (Perry *et al.*, 1978), any therapeutic intervention that fails to address the cholinergic loss is unlikely to be totally effective.

Furthermore, the restoration of cholinergic tone in the hippocampus may be particularly important because in some demented patients cholinergic loss may be confined to this area (Bowen et al., 1979; Rossor et al., 1984) and because of the critical involvement of the temporal lobes in memory function. Of course, in addition to the technical problems associated with fetal tissue tranplantation there are considerable ethical and medico-legal issues to be confronted (Hoffer & Olson, 1991) and it may be that other transplantation strategies will be developed to overcome these difficulties. Such strategies might include the transplantation of transfected cells carrying genes that express trophic factors (e.g. nerve growth factor) or enzymes that are required for the production of relevant neurotransmitters (e.g. tyrosine hydroxylase). Experiments using such techniques in animals have already produced encouraging results (Fischer et al., 1987; Freed et al., 1990; Gage et al., 1990; Horellou et al., 1990).

References

Annett, L. E., Dunnett, S. B., Martel, F. L. et al. (1990). A functional assessment of embryonic dopaminergic grafts in the marmoset. Progress in Brain Research, **82**, 535–42.

Arendt, T., Allen, Y., Sinden, J. et al. (1988). Cholinergic-rich brain transplants reverse alcohol-induced memory deficits. Nature, **332**, 448–50.

Arendt, T., Bigl, V., Arendt, A. & Tennstedt, A. (1983). Loss of neurons in the nucleus basalis of Meynert in Alzheimer's disease, paralysis agitans and Korsakoff's disease. Acta Neuropathologica, **61**, 101–8.

Backlund, E. O., Granberg, P. O., Hamberger, B. et al. (1985). Transplantation of adrenal medullary tissue to striatum in parkinsonism. First clinical trials. Journal of Neurosurgery, **62**, 169–73.

Bakay, R. A. E., Barrow, D. L., Fiandaca, M. S. et al. (1987) Biochemical and behavioral correction of MPTP parkinsonian-like syndrome by fetal cell transplantation. Annals New York Academy of Sciences, **495**, 623–40.

Bankiewicz, K. S., Plunkett, R. J., Mefford, I. et al. (1990). Behavioral recovery from MPTP-induced parkinsonism in monkeys after intracerebral tissue implants is not related to CSF concentrations of dopamine metabolites. Progress in Brain Research, **82**, 561–71.

Björklund, A., Dunnett, S. B., Stenevi, U. et al. (1980). Reinnervation of the denervated striatum by substantia nigra transplants: functional consequences as revealed by pharmacological and sensorimotor testing. Brain Research, **199**, 307–33.

Björklund, A., Lindvall, O., Isacson, O. et al. (1987). Mechanisms of action of intracerebral neural implants. Trends in Neurosciences, **10**, 509–16.

Björklund, A. & Stenevi, U. (1977). Reformation of the severed septohippocampal pathway in the adult rat by transplanted septal neurons. Cell Tissue Research, **185**, 289–302.

Björklund, A. & Stenevi, U. (1979). Reconstruction of the nigrostriatal dopamine pathway by intracerebral nigral transplants. Brain Research, **177**, 555–60.

Bondareff, W., Mountjoy, C. Q. & Roth, M. (1981). Selective loss of neurones of origin of adrenergic projection to cerebral cortex (nucleus locus coeruleus) in senile dementia. Lancet, **i**, 783–4.

Bowen, D. M., Smith, C. B., White, P. & Davison, A. N. (1976). Neurotransmitter-related enzymes and indices of hypoxia in senile dementia and other abiotrophies. *Brain*, **99**, 459–96.

Bowen, D. M., White, P., Spillane, J. A. *et al.* (1979). Accelerated ageing or selective neuronal loss as an important cause of dementia? *Lancet*, **i**, 11–14.

Clarke, D. J., Gage, F. H. & Björklund, A. (1986). Formation of cholinergic synapses by intrahippocampal septal grafts as revealed by choline acetyltransferase immunocytochemistry. *Brain Research*, **369**, 151–62.

Clarke, D. J., Nilsson, O. G., Brundin, P. & Bjorklund, A. (1990). Synaptic connections formed by grafts of different types of cholinergic neurons in the host hippocampus. *Experimental Neurology*, **107**, 11–22.

Cross, A. J., Crow, T. J., Perry, E. K. *et al.* (1981). Reduced dopamine-beta-hydroxylase activity in Alzheimer's disease. *British Medical Journal*, **282**, 93–4.

Das, G. D. & Altman, J. (1971). Transplanted precursors of nerve cells: their fate in the cerebellums of young rats. *Science*, **173**, 637–8.

Davies, P. & Maloney, A. J. (1976). Selective loss of central cholinergic neurones in Alzheimer's disease. *Lancet*, **ii**, 1430.

Dunnett, S. B. (1990). Neural transplantation in animal models of dementia. *European Journal of Neuroscience*, **2**, 567–87.

Dunnett, S. B., Björklund, A., Schmidt, R. H. *et al.* (1983). Intracerebral grafting of neuronal cell suspensions. IV Behavioural recovery in rats with unilateral 6-OHDA lesions following implantation of nigral cell suspensions in different forebrain sites. *Acta Physiologica Scandinavica* (Suppl.), **522**, 29–37.

Dunnett, S. B., Low, W. C., Iversen, S. D. *et al.* (1982). Septal transplants restore maze learning in rats with fornix-fimbria lesions. *Brain Research*, **251**, 335–48.

Fibiger, H. C. (1991). Cholinergic mechanisms in learning, memory and dementia: a review of recent evidence. *Trends in Neurosciences*, **14**, 220–3.

Fine, A. (1990). Transplantation of adrenal tissue into the central nervous system. *Brain Research Reviews*, **15**, 121–33.

Fine A., Hunt, S. P., Oertel, W. H. *et al.* (1988). Transplantation of embryonic marmoset dopaminergic neurons to the corpus striatum of marmosets rendered parkinsonian by 1-methyl-4-phenyl-1,2,3,6-tetrahydropyridine. *Progress in Brain Research*, **78**, 479–89.

Fischer, W., Wictorin, K., Björklund, A. *et al.* (1987). Amelioration of cholinergic neuron atrophy and spatial memory impairment in aged rats by nerve growth factor. *Nature*, **329**, 65–8.

Freed, W. J., Geller, H. M., Poltorak, M. *et al.* (1990). Genetically altered and defined cell lines for transplantation in animal models of Parkinson's disease. *Progress in Brain Research*, **82**, 11–21.

Freed, C. R., Richards, J. B., Sabol, K. E. & Reite, M. L. (1988). Fetal substantia nigra transplants lead to dopamine cell replacement and behavioural improvement in bonnet monkeys with MPTP induced parkinsonism. In *Pharmacology and functional regulation of dopaminergic neurons*. (ed. P. M. Beart, G. N. Woodruff & D. M. Jackson), pp. 353–60. MacMillan, London.

Gage, F. H., Björklund, A., Stenevi, U. *et al.* (1984). Intrahippocampal septal grafts ameliorate learning deficits in aged rats. *Science*, **225**, 533–6.

Gage, F. H., Fisher, L. J., Jinnah, H. A. *et al.* (1990). Grafting genetically modified cells to the brain: conceptual and technical issues. *Progress Brain Research*, **82**, 1–9.

Garcia-Flores, E., Decanini, H. L., Flores Salazar, M. *et al.* (1990). Is autologous transplant of adrenal medulla ino the striatum an effective therapy for Parkinson's disease? *Progress in Brain Research*, **82**, 643–55.

Hitchcock, E. R., Kenny, B. G., Clough, C. G. *et al.* (1990). Stereotactic implantation of foetal mesencephalon (STIM). *Progress in Brain Research*, **82**, 723–30.

Hodges, H., Allen, Y., Sinden, J. *et al.* (1990). Cholinergic-rich transplants alleviate cognitive deficits in lesioned rats, but exacerbate response to cholinergic drugs. *Progress in Brain Research*, **82**, 347–58.

Hoffer, B. J. & Olson, L. (1991). Ethical issues in brain cell transplantation. *Trends in Neurosciences*, **14**, 384–8.

Horellou, P., Marlier, L., Privat, A. *et al.* (1990). Exogeneous expression of L-DOPA and dopamine in various cell lines following transfer of rat and human tyrosine hydroxylase cDNA: grafting in an animal model of Parkinson's disease. *Progress in Brain Research*, **82**, 23–32.

Lieberman, A., Ransohoff, J., Berczeller, P. & Goldstein, M. (1990). Adrenal medullary transplants as a treatment for advanced Parkinson's disease. *Progressive Brain Research*, **82**, 665–70.

Lindvall, O., Backlund, E. O., Farde L. *et al.* (1987). Transplantation in Parkinson's disease: two cases of adrenal medullary grafts to the putamen. *Annals of Neurology*, **22**, 457–68.

Lindvall, O. & Björklund, A. (1989). Transplantation strategies in the treatment of Parkinson's disease: experimental basis and clinical trials. *Acta Neurologica Scandinavica*, **126**, 197–210.

Lindvall, O., Brundin, P., Widner, H. *et al.* (1990). Grafts of fetal dopamine neurons survive and improve motor function in Parkinson's disease. *Science*, **247**, 574–7.

Lindvall, O., Rehncrona, S., Brundin, P. *et al.* (1989). Human fetal dopamine neurons grafted into the striatum in two patients with severe Parkinson's disease. *Archives of Neurology*, **46**, 615–31.

Low, W. C., Lewis, P. R., Bunch, S. T. *et al.* (1982). Function recovery following neural transplantation of embryonic septal nuclei in adult rats with septohippo-campal lesions. *Nature*, **300**, 260–2.

Madrazo, I., Drucker-Colin, R., Diaz, V. *et al.* (1987). Open microsurgical autograft of adrenal medulla to the right caudate nucleus in two patients with intractable Parkinson's disease. *New England Journal of Medicine*, **316**, 831–4.

Madrazo, I., Franco-Bourland, R., Aguilera, M. & Ostrosky-Solis, F. (1989). Hispanic registry of graft procedure for Parkinson's disease. *Lancet*, **2**, 751–2.

Madrazo, I., Leon, V., Torres, C. *et al.* (1988). Transplantation of fetal substantia nigra and adrenal medulla to the caudate nucleus in two patients with Parkinson's disease. *New England Journal of Medicine*, **318**, 51.

Nakano, I. & Hirano, A. (1982). Loss of large neurons of the medial septal nucleus in an autopsy case of Alzheimer's disease. *Journal of Neuropathology and Experimental Neurology*, **41**, 341.

Nilsson, O. G., Kalen, P., Rosengren, E. & Björklund, A. (1990). Acetylcholine release from intrahippocampal septal grafts is under control of the host brain. *Proceedings of the National Academy of Sciences*, **87**, 2647–51.

Perlow, M. J., Freed, W. J., Hoffer, B. J. *et al.* (1979). Brain grafts reduce motor abnormalities produced by destruction of the nigrostriatal dopamine system. *Science*, **204**, 643–7.

Perry, E. K., Curtis, M., Dick, D. J. *et al.* (1985). Cholinergic correlates of cognitive impairment in Parkinson's disease: comparison with Alzheimer's disease. *Journal of Neurology, Neurosurgery and Psychiatry*, **48**, 413–21.

Perry, E. K., Gibson, P. H., Blessed, G. *et al.* (1977). Neurotransmitter enzyme abnormalities in senile dementia. *Journal of Neurological Sciences*, **34**, 247–65.

Perry, E. K., Tomlinson, B. E., Blessed, G. *et al.* (1978). Correlation of cholinergic abnormalities with senile plaques and mental test scores in senile dementia. *British Medical Journal*, **2**, 1457–9.

Ridley, R. M. & Baker, H. F. (1991). A critical evaluation of monkey models of amnesia and dementia. *Brain Research Reviews*, **16**, 15–37.

Ridley, R. M., Murray, T. K., Johnson, J. A. & Baker, H. F. (1986). Learning impairment following lesion of the basal nucleus of Meynert in the marmoset: modification by cholinergic drugs. *Brain Research*, **376**, 108–16.

Ridley, R. M., Thornley, H. D., Baker, H. F. & Fine, A. (1991). Cholinergic neural transplants into hippocampus restore learning ability in monkeys with fornix transections. *Experimental Brain Research*, **83**, 533–8.

Ridley, R. M., Samson, N. A., Baker, H. F. & Johnson, J. A. (1988). Visuospatial learning impairment following lesion of the cholinergic projection to the hippocampus. *Brain Research*, **456**, 71–87.

Roberts, G. W., Crow, T. J. & Polak, J. M. (1985). Location of neuronal tangles in somatostatin neurones in Alzheimer's disease. *Nature*, **314**, 92–4.

Rossor, M. N., Iversen, L. L., Reynolds, G. P. *et al.* (1984). Neurochemical characteristics of early and late onset types of Alzheimer's disease. *British Medical Journal*, **288**, 961–4.

Schmidt, R. H., Björklund, A. & Stenevi, U. (1981). Intracerebral grafting of dissociated CNS tissue suspensions: new approach for neuronal transplantation to deep brain sites. *Brain Research*, **218**, 347–56.

Taylor, J. R., Elsworth, J. D., Roth, R. H. *et al.* (1990). Improvements in MPTP-induced object retrieval deficits and behavioural deficits after fetal nigral grafting in monkeys. *Progress in Brain Research*, **82**, 543–59.

Whitehouse, P. J., Price, D. L., Struble, R. G. *et al.* (1982). Alzheimer's disease and senile dementia: loss of neurones in the basal forebrain. *Science*, **215**, 1237–9.

Note added in proof

A more recent account of the effects of dopamine-rich grafts in the basal ganglia of marmosets with unilateral 6-OHDA lesions is given by Annett (1994) and Annett *et al.* (1994).

We have now demonstrated that acetylcholine-rich tissue grafted into the neocortex of primates with damage to cortical cholinergic projections can produce substantial restitution of function (Ridley *et al.*, 1994).

A recent review of human transplant cases is given by Lindvall (1994).

Annett, L. E. (1994). Function studies of neural grafts in parkinsonian primates. In *Functional neural transplantation* (ed. S. B. Dunnett & A. Björklund), pp. 71–102. Raven Press Ltd., New York.

Annett, L. E., Martel, F. L., Rogers, D. C. *et al.* (1994). Behavioral assessment of the effects of embryonic nigral grafts in marmosets with unilateral 6-OHDA lesions of the nigrostriatal pathway. *Experimental Neurology*, **125**, 228–46.

Lindvall, O. (1994). Neural transplantation in Parkinson's disease. In *Functional neural transplantation* (ed. S. B. Dunnett & A. Björklund), pp. 71–102. Raven Press Ltd., New York.

Ridley, R. M., Baker, J. A., Baker, H. F. & Maclean, C. J. (1994). Restoration of cognitive abilities by cholinergic grafts in cortex of monkeys with lesions of the basal nucleus of Meynert. *Neuroscience*, **63**, 653–66.

10

Methods of construction of transgenic animals and applications of the technology

FRANCES BUSFIELD, KAREN DUFF, CORINNE LENDON and ALISON GOATE

A number of techniques have been developed over the last decade to allow the introduction of defined DNA sequences into the germline of mice and other mammals. Once inserted, these sequences, termed transgenes, are stably transmitted from generation to generation. The transgene may be expressed, although not always, and subjected to the correct developmental, tissue specific and physiological regulation.

Why make transgenic animals?

As methods for the production of transgenic animals are refined so that the expression pattern of the transgene is more predictable, the applications of the technique have become more widespread. Transgenic animals can be used to study various aspects of gene expression and regulation, and more recently to develop animal models of human disease. Preliminary studies to identify regulatory elements of a gene can be carried out *in vitro* by the use of transient transfection assays. However, transfection studies in cultured cells will not identify elements required for tissue-specific expression if it is not possible to culture a specific cell type, or identify elements required for temporal expression of developmentally regulated genes. Such questions can only be addressed through transgenic experiments.

With the recent development of gene targeting we now have the potential to generate mice of any desired genotype. This has enabled the construction of null mutants, i.e. mice with no functioning gene at a given locus, and mouse models of human genetic disease. The ability to choose how to mutate a gene will allow a thorough analysis of function of any cloned gene through the analysis of multiple mutant alleles and should greatly facilitate the analysis of complex processes such as mammalian development.

Methods for the construction of transgenic animals

The most commonly used animal for transgenic experiments is the mouse (Palmiter & Brinster, 1986). However, rats, sheep, goats, pigs and cattle are being used for some studies. Three different protocols are currently used for the production of transgenic mice: recombinant retroviral infection (Jaenisch, 1976), microinjection of DNA (Brinster *et al.*, 1981) and gene targeting in embryonic stem cells (Capecchi, 1989). The protocols will be discussed in the order in which they were developed.

Infection of preimplantation embryos with recombinant retroviruses

Retroviral infection is achieved by co-cultivation of embryos stripped of their zona pellucida and fibroblasts producing recombinant virus (Jaenisch *et al.*, 1981; Jahner *et al.*, 1985; van der Putten *et al.*, 1985; Hogan, Costantini & Lacy, 1986). Blastocysts are then reimplanted into pseudopregnant mice. Retroviral integration occurs via a precise mechanism, which results in the insertion of a single, intact copy of the provirus containing the gene of interest flanked by retroviral LTRs. However, although each integration event is single copy, multiple events can occur in each cell of the embryo. The founder animals are therefore mosaic for many insertions. The frequency of integration is high but germline transmission is low because of the mosaicism, which requires extensive outbreeding to establish pure breeding lines showing Mendelian transmission (Jaenisch *et al.*, 1981; van der Putten *et al.*, 1985). The heterozygotes for single proviral integration events can then be bred to produce mice homozygous for the foreign gene.

This was the first protocol established for the introduction of foreign DNA into the mouse germline and has the advantages of being technically simple to carry out and does not require any expensive equipment. The retroviral construct can also be introduced into post-implantation embryos or into specific tissues. The retrovirus provides a marker for cell lineage experiments. The disadvantages of this technique include: (1) the need to clone your gene of interest into a viral vector that can be transfected into a helper cell line producing specific infectious recombinant viral particles; (2) the piece of DNA to be inserted into the retrovirus must be less than 10 kb; (3) the effect of strong viral regulatory elements contained within the LTRs upon the specificity of the expression of the transgene is unknown; (4) the chromosomal site of integration may interfere with efficient expression of the transgene (Jaenisch *et al.*, 1981).

Microinjection of foreign DNA into one-cell mouse embryos

A general scheme for the production of transgenic animals using this method is shown in Figure 10.1 (Hogan *et al.*, 1986; Palmiter & Brinster, 1986; Allen *et al.*, 1987). Donor female mice are superovulated and mated with a stud male mouse. Twelve hours post coitum the female mice are sacrificed, the oviducts are removed and fertilized one-cell embryos are harvested and placed in culture. 1–2 pl of purified cloned DNA fragment, at 1–2 ng/ml, is then

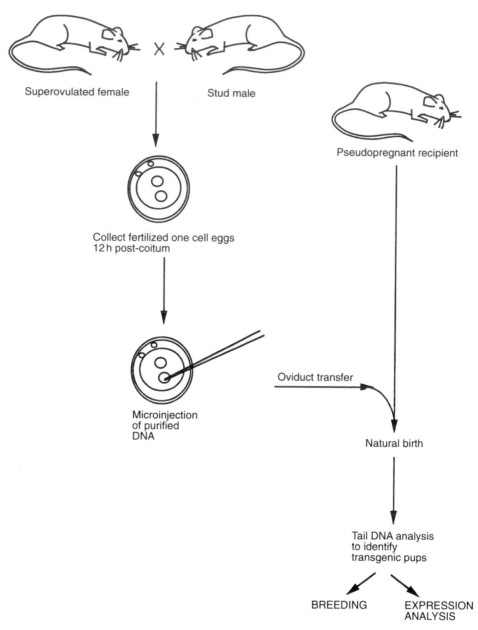

Figure 10.1. Schematic diagram of transgenic mouse production by microinjection of DNA into the pronucleus of one-cell embryos.

microinjected into the pronucleus of the embryo; this gives an optimal DNA integration frequency of 20–40% (Brinster *et al.*, 1985). The embryos are placed in an incubator for several hours to recover, then transferred into the oviduct of a pseudopregnant female mouse. Transgenic pups are identified in the litter by clipping the end of the tail, extracting DNA and either carrying out

PCR or Southern blots. Transgenic animals are then bred to establish a breeding colony for each transgenic line. These animals can then be used for expression analysis.

Exogenous DNA, in all cells, is carried by 80% of transgenic mice, indicating that the foreign DNA integrated prior to the first round of DNA replication. However, in 20% of cases the foreign DNA integrates after the first round of replication, leading to mosaic animals in which the proportion of transgenic offspring depends upon the proportion of germ cells containing the transgene (Costantini & Lacy, 1981).

The foreign DNA integrates into the mouse genome at random. The copy number of transgenes can vary considerably (one to several hundred) depending on the concentration of DNA injected. Single-copy integration events can be favoured by lowering the concentration of DNA to be injected, however this strategy must be balanced by the necessity to inject a larger number of eggs, owing to the drop in overall integration efficiency (Chada *et al.*, 1985). Multiple copies of the transgene invariably have a single site of insertion tandemly arranged head to tail (Brinster *et al.*, 1981; Costantini & Lacy, 1981).

The efficiency of this technique varies depending on the skill of those carrying out the experiments. However, rough estimates of the efficiency of each stage are that 60–80% of embryos survive microinjection, 10–30% of embryos implant and develop normally and 10–30% of pups are transgenic (Hogan *et al.*, 1986). Linear DNA integrates into the mouse genome five-fold more efficiently than supercoiled DNA (Brinster *et al.*, 1985). Removal of vector sequences from the construct also increases the chances of expression of the construct one thousand-fold (Chada *et al.*, 1985; Townes *et al.*, 1985). The strain of mouse used affects the efficiency, as does the dexterity of the person carrying out the microinjection.

The biggest disadvantage of this technique is that many transgenic animals do not express their transgene unless a great deal of work has been carried out to identify sequences required for site-independent temporal and spatial expression of the gene under study. If a weak heterologous promoter or insufficient sequences from the endogenous promoter are included in the construct, then vector sequences or the site of chromosomal integration may affect gene expression. Either expression may reflect a fraction of the normal level or inappropriate spatial or temporal expression may occur. The extent and location of sequences required for the appropriate expression varies considerably: elastase and γ-crystallin genes only require a few hundred base pairs 5′ to the coding sequence (Swift & Hammer, 1984; Goring *et al.*, 1987); alphafetoprotein requires 10 kb of sequence 5′ to the coding sequence (Hammer *et al.*, 1987) and α-globin requires sequences both 5′ and 3′ to the coding sequence (Trudel & Costantini, 1987).

In small genes, such as the prion protein gene in which the entire coding sequence is in a single exon, microinjection of a genomic clone (cosmid) containing the gene and flanking sequences appears to produce the correct expression pattern (Scott *et al.*, 1989; Hsiao *et al.*, 1990). The main problem arising from this method is therefore correct gene expression, particularly when the gene under study is encoded by many exons covering more than 50 kb of genomic DNA, since cDNA clones then have to be used for the construct with either a heterologous promoter or with endogenous sequences spliced onto the 5' end of the cDNA. The need to know the structure of the promoter could be overcome if the gene was inserted at the correct position in the genome by homologous recombination. However, in the mouse genome only 1/1000 integration events are by homologous recombination (Thomas & Capecchi, 1987). The development of *in vitro* techniques for selection of homologous recombinants has now made this a feasible approach.

Gene targeting in embryonic stem (ES) cells

Gene targeting has the potential to generate mice of any desired genotype (Capecchi, 1989). Specific mutations are generated in a cloned DNA sequence from the desired locus using recombinant DNA techniques. The mutation is then transferred via homologous recombination (HR) to the genome of embryonic stem (ES) cells (Doetschman *et al.*, 1987; Thomas & Capecchi, 1987). ES cells are pluripotent cells, derived from the inner cell mass of blastocysts, which can be cultured and manipulated *in vitro* (Evans & Kaufman, 1981; Martin, 1981). When injected into a blastocyst, ES cells colonize the embryo, participating in normal development and contributing to all somatic tissues and germ cells (Robertson *et al.*, 1986). A construct can therefore be introduced into ES cells and homologous recombinants selected *in vitro* before injection into blastocysts. Founder animals are chimaeras and must be bred to produce animals heterozygous for the targeted gene (Bradley *et al.*, 1984). Sometimes ES cells fail to colonize the germline, probably due to the accumulation of chromosomal abnormalities whilst in culture. It is therefore extremely important to look after the cells whilst they are in culture, to use early-passage cells and to have them karyotyped frequently.

Several methods for the selection of homologous recombinants have now been developed (Capecchi, 1989). Figure 10.2 shows a general protocol for the production of transgenic animals using gene targeting. The majority of gene targeting experiments carried out so far have involved gene disruption in order to create null mutants (Mansour, Thomas & Capecchi, 1988; Joyner, Skarnes & Rossant, 1989; Schwartzberg, Goff & Robertson, 1989; Zimmer & Gruss, 1989; McMahon & Bradley, 1990). However, the procedure does have the potential to create subtle mutations (Hasty *et al.*, 1991*a*). The design of construct depends very much on the purpose of the experiment.

Male ES cells are electroporated in the presence of the targeting construct. Cells are then grown in the presence of G418 (a neomycin analogue) to select

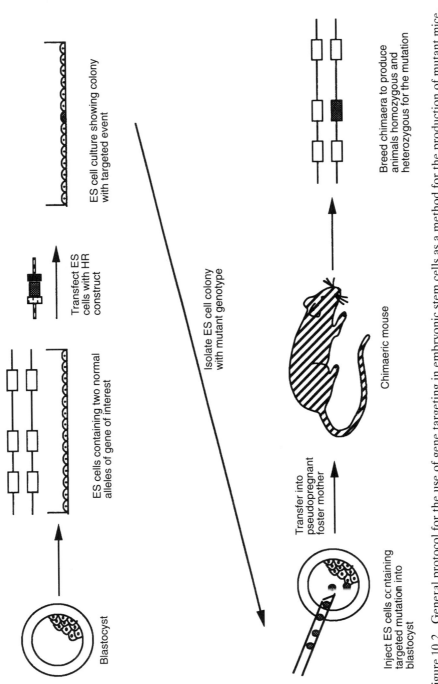

ES cell culture showing colony
with targeted event

Transfect ES
cells with HR
construct

ES cells containing two normal
alleles of gene of interest

Isolate ES cell colony
with mutant genotype

Breed chimaera to produce
animals homozygous and
heterozygous for the mutation

Chimaeric mouse

Transfer into
pseudopregnant
foster mother

Blastocyst

Inject ES cells containing
targeted mutation into
blastocyst

Figure 10.2. General protocol for the use of gene targeting in embryonic stem cells as a method for the production of mutant mice.

for cells that have taken up the targeting construct (positive selection). The second selection then enriches for homologous recombinants, in one of several ways. For a small proportion of genes, direct selection is possible if the ES line is negative for the gene, e.g. HPRT (Doetschman et al., 1987; Thomas & Capecchi, 1987). Direct PCR screening of all clones using primers that will amplify only if the construct has integrated via HR has been used for several genes (Kim & Smithies, 1988; Joyner et al., 1989; Zimmer & Gruss, 1989). Depending on the frequency of HR, this may necessitate using PCR to test anywhere from several hundred to several thousand clones. If the gene to be targeted is expressed in ES cells then promoterless neomycin constructs can be used so that the first selection enriches for integration events occurring in expressed sequences. PCR screening of these clones should give some enrichment over the first procedure (Jasin & Berg, 1988). Only minimal expression of the target gene in embryonic stem cells is required to enrich for homologous recombinants using promoterless vectors (Jeannotte, Ruiz & Robertson, 1991). Another widely applicable method is the incorporation of a gene such as herpes simplex virus thymidine kinase (HSV-tk) within the HR construct beyond the region of homology with the mouse genome, so that the gene will not be integrated into the genome if homologous recombination occurs. Addition of ganciclovir (a drug with selective sensitivity for cells expressing herpes simplex thymidine kinase) to the ES cells will result in the death of those in which the construct integrated at random, since HSV-tk will be expressed (negative selection) (Mansour et al., 1988; McMahon & Bradley, 1990). This technique is not 100% effective but has been shown to enrich for HR with several different constructs. Several parameters are known to affect the frequency of homologous recombination, including the length of the regions of homology and non-homology and the availability of free ends (Hasty, Rivera-Perez & Bradley, 1991b; Hasty et al., 1991c). Insertion vectors target more frequently than replacement vectors. Both types of vector require a critical length of homology for maximum targeting efficiency, e.g. a dramatic increase in absolute targeting efficiency was observed at the hprt locus when the length of homology was increased from 1.3 to 6.8 kb. A detailed discussion of the considerations necessary in construct design may be found elsewhere (Capecchi, 1989; McMahon & Bradley, 1990; Hasty et al., 1991b, c).

Gene targeting enables recessive lethals to be maintained as heterozygotes. It has the potential to create mouse models of human genetic disease. The caveat to this is that differences in the metabolism of proteins between man and mouse mean that the disease phenotype may not always be reproduced in the mouse. HPRT (hypoxanthine phosphoribosyl transferase) deficiency in humans causes Lesch–Nyhan syndrome but in mice there is no clearly discernible abnormal phenotype (Koller et al., 1989). The mdx mouse produces only 10% of normal levels of dystrophin transcripts but does not appear to suffer from the severe muscle wasting associated with defects at the homologous locus in man (Duchenne and Becker muscular dystrophies). This would appear to be due to the fact that the *mdx* mouse is capable of regenerating muscle, which does not happen in the human diseases.

The application of transgenic technologies

Gene expression

Transgenic animals can be used to study various aspects of gene expression and regulation. A commonly used strategy is to construct hybrid genes in which the control elements from the gene of interest are used to direct the expression of a 'reporter' gene. Reporter gene constructs can be used to determine which regulatory elements are required for the correct temporal and spatial pattern of the gene under study. Two of the most commonly used reporter genes are the bacterial chloramphenicol acetyl transferase (CAT) and β-galactosidase (*lacZ*) genes. Using either of these reporter genes, a series of constructs can be made that contain overlapping fragments of the putative promoter sequences spliced 5' to the reporter gene. The role of splicing in the regulation of gene expression has been assessed by the generation of transgenic mice carrying the histone H4 promoter linked to the CAT gene with or without heterologous introns within the transcription unit (Choi *et al.*, 1991).

A series of constructs can be made containing overlapping fragments of a putative promoter sequence spliced 5' to the coding sequence for *lacZ*. If the sequence induces *lacZ* expression this can be detected histochemically either in whole mouse embryos or in tissue sections. β-Galactosidase hydrolyses lactose to produce galactose and glucose. When 5-bromo-4-chloro-3-indolyl-β-D-galactoside (X-gal) is provided as a substrate for β-galactosidase *in vitro* it is cleaved to produce a chromogenic (blue) product. The expression pattern of β-galactosidase can then be compared with the pattern of expression of the endogenous gene from which the putative promoter sequences are derived. Analysis of a number of different genes has demonstrated that regulatory elements may be present up to 50 kb from the coding sequence of a gene and can lie either 5' or 3' to the gene or in introns within the gene. This approach has been used to test whether the putative promoter regions of the amyloid precursor protein gene, Thy-1 and neurone-specific enolase, identified via CAT assays *in vitro*, drive neurone-specific transcription *in vivo* (Gordon *et al.*, 1987; Forss-Petter *et al.*, 1990; Wirak *et al.*, 1991*a*).

A second strategy for the identification of regulatory sequences is the use of 'tagging' the transgene. This can be done either by incorporating DNA from a different species (Meyer *et al.*, 1990), by using a Minigene with some of the exons deleted, or modifying the gene by insertion or deletion of a few nucleotides to insert a specific antigenic determinant recognized by a mono-clonal antibody. This strategy can be employed when the levels of expression are to be assayed and quantified to show that the transgene is being expressed at the correct levels and in the correct tissues. Several of these tagging methods were employed in a study into the effect of introns on transcriptional efficiency. The level of expression of intron-containing and intronless genes was compared for three genes. Two of these genes were from a different species and their expression was easily distinguished from that of the endogenous mouse genes. The third gene was the mouse metallothionein I gene, which was oligonucleotide marked in order to distinguish its expression from that of the endogenous metallothionein gene (Brinster *et al.*, 1988; Palmiter *et al.*, 1991).

These strategies are relatively straightforward if only a single element is involved, but may be very complicated where several elements act in a redundant or co-operative manner. Transgenic mice have also been used extensively in the study of developmentally important genes. Expression of the β-globin genes has been the subject of intense investigation in transgenic mice. The recent discovery of the locus control region (LCR) and the information from transgenic experiments has provided new insight into the molecular control of globin gene switching (Raich *et al.*, 1990; Shih, Wall & Shapiro, 1990; Stamatoyannopoulos, 1991). During development, the expression of the human globin gene switches from embryonic (ε and δ) in the yolk sac to fetal (γ) during interuterine life to adult (β) after birth. Experiments in transgenic mice have suggested at least two mechanisms are involved in the developmental control of globin gene switching, an autonomous mode in the embryonic gene (Raich *et al.*, 1990) and a competitive mode as illustrated by the switch from fetal to adult globin gene expression (Shih *et al.*, 1990; Stamatoyannopoulos, 1991).

Aberrant expression of transgenes in a particular transgenic mouse line is often attributed to chromosomal position effects. Transgenes showing aberrant expression have now been isolated and reintroduced into the mouse genome to produce secondary transgenic mice that show a normal expression pattern, indicating that the position of transgene insertion can affect its expression (Al-Shawi *et al.*, 1990). This is probably due to the presence of strong control elements nearby, which influence the expression of the transgene; chromosomal domains that influence developmental expression can therefore be identified using transgenes that integrate randomly throughout the genome. Positional effects are exerted most strongly in transgenes that contain a weak promoter, e.g. the herpes simplex virus thymidine kinase promoter and no other modulating sequences.

Mammalian development

When constructs are made that have a weak promoter linked to a reporter gene such as *lacZ*, they can be used as an enhancer trap to identify chromosomal domains active during development (Allen *et al.*, 1988; Kothary *et al.*, 1988; Gossler *et al.*, 1989). *LacZ* expression will occur only if the construct has integrated into the genome within an expressed gene in the correct reading frame. Since the transgene is transmitted to subsequent generations, a systematic analysis of its expression during development is possible. If *lacZ* is expressed in a spatially or temporally restricted manner, reflecting some specific developmental control, then the sequences surrounding the integration site can easily be cloned to identify genes involved in mammalian development. Breeding of these transgenic lines to produce animals homozygous for the gene disruption frequently leads to abnormal phenotypes. In several cases, insertion of a transgene has led to a phenotype identical to a known spontaneous mutation in the mouse (Woychik *et al.*, 1985; Kothary *et al.*, 1988). Subsequent mapping of the site of integration and crossing of animals heterozygous for each mutation has demonstrated that they are allelic variants.

Insertion mutagenesis (gene trap) has also been used to identify loci critical for normal development, i.e. random insertion of a piece of DNA that causes an abnormal phenotype through disruption of the gene at the site of insertion (Jaenisch, 1976; Woychik *et al.*, 1985). These experiments have been carried out using both recombinant retroviruses and DNA microinjection. Cloning the sequences at the site of integration is relatively easy if the gene has been inactivated by a retrovirus, particularly if it has been tagged with a suppressor gene to allow selection in *E. coli*. The first embryonic lethal insertional mutation characterized is the *Mov-13* retrovirally induced mutation, which disrupts the $\alpha1(I)$ collagen gene. Continued accumulation of insertional mutations may identify important developmental genes. However, this is a serendipitous approach and therefore not ideal as a screening procedure for the identification of specific mutations.

Transgenic animals provide models to study the activities of genes and their protein products whose complex molecular biology in the whole body would otherwise be difficult to interpret. The molecular mechanisms of parental imprinting have been studied in transgenic animals due to the serendipitous integration of a *c-myc* transgene into a region of DNA, which when inherited from the male is expressed in the heart. It is not expressed at any stage during development if inherited from the female. Their results support the hypothesis that the parental origin of certain genes governs their degree of methylation and therefore determines their expression (Swain, Stewart & Leder, 1987).

The study of cell lineage and cell fate has provided an important tool for understanding development. Several methods have traditionally been used to carry out cell ablation, including the removal of cells by microdissection or laser irradiation. *LacZ* reporter gene constructs have also been used to visualize lineage-specific gene expression. In mammals, these studies have been extended through the use of promoter or enhancer directed ablation of specific cell lineages by coupling expression of a cytotoxic gene product to tissue-specific promoters (Palmiter *et al.*, 1987). Cell death has most commonly been affected by expression of the A chain of diphtheria toxin (DT-A). DT-A encodes an adenine diphosphate (ADP) ribosyltransferase that inhibits protein synthesis by catalysing the ADP ribosylation of elongation factor 2. DT-A is unable to enter the cell in the absence of the diphtheria toxin B chain, and is therefore limited to the cell in which it has been expressed under the control of the exogenous promoter.

The specifity of cell ablation is achieved by coupling the toxin gene to the promoter of a gene that is expressed in only one cell type. One such gene encodes the elastase 1 polypeptide, the synthesis of which is restricted to the acinar cells of the pancreas. Microinjection of a construct consisting of the elastase 1 promoter/enhancer fused to the coding region of the DT-A gene generated transgenic mice lacking a normal pancreas, owing to ablation of the pancreatic acinar cells (Palmiter et al., 1987). A second gene, γ-crystallin, is restricted to the terminally differentiated fibre cells of the lens. Transgenic mice microinjected with the DT-A coding region used to the γ2-crystallin promoter underwent ablation of this cell type and showed a high incidence of microphthalmia (Breitman et al., 1987). Cell type ablation is therefore a powerful method for investigating developmental lineages, especially where the cells' contribution to organogenesis is unknown.

Genetic ablation of specific genes can now be achieved using gene targeting. Indeed, null mutations have now been created in a number of important developmentally regulated genes (Mansour et al., 1988; Joyner et al., 1989; Schwartzberg et al., 1989; Zimmer & Gruss, 1989; McMahon & Bradley, 1990). The phenotype of such a mouse may give clues to the function of a specific protein and identify tissues or cell types in which the protein is required for normal development. Surprisingly, some of the homeo-box containing genes, which might have been expected to produce embryonic lethal pheno-types when knocked-out, give subtly different phenotypes with no apparent detriment to the organism. This may be because these genes are members of large gene families in which there may be some redundancy.

Models of human genetic disease

Putative disease-causing mutations identified through human molecular gene-tics can be tested in mice to determine whether they are pathogenic. For small genes, such as the prion protein gene (PrP), which is encoded in a single exon, microinjection of a linearized cosmid produces the normal pattern of gene expression (Scott et al., 1989; Hsiao et al., 1990; Prusiner et al., 1990). Insertion of a point mutation, observed in the human population, that is thought to lead to Gerstmann–Sträussler–Scheinker syndrome (GSS), into the homologous codon in a mouse PrP cosmid results in mice that develop spontaneous neurodegenerative disease with a phenotype very similar to GSS (Hsiao et al., 1990). Construction of transgenic mice containing PrP genes from hamster, followed by challenge of these animals with prion inoculum from both hamster and mouse brains, has contributed greatly to our understanding of the mechanisms involved in these transmissible dementias (Scott et al., 1989; Prusiner et al., 1990). The use of DNA microinjection as a method of producing transgenics is more problematic when the gene of interest is encoded by many exons covering more than 50 kb of genomic DNA. This is because genomic clones cannot, at present, be used for the constructs. Instead, hybrid constructs have to be made between cDNA clones and either heterologous or autologous promoter sequences. This may result in an aberrant pattern of gene expression or very low levels of expression (Palmiter & Brinster, 1986). Several labs are at present trying to develop techniques to transfect or microinject cells with yeast artificial chromosomes (YACs), which will allow the introduction of much larger pieces of foreign genomic DNA (several hundreds of kb) (Reeves, Pavan & Hieter, 1990). In disorders such as Alzheimer's disease, where overexpression of the normal gene is predicted to cause the pathology, DNA microinjection of one-cell embryos cannot easily be used to test putative disease-causing mutations since the copy number of the gene will be increased. Indeed, several transgenic mouse lines have now been created that develop a neuropathology similar to AD by overexpressing normal human APP or fragments of normal human APP (Kawabata, Higgins & Gordon, 1991; Quon *et al.*, 1991; Wirak *et al.*, 1991*b*).

In addition to the creation of null mutants, gene targeting techniques enable the creation of subtle mutations that may affect structure, function or regulation of a protein (Capecchi, 1989; Hasty *et al.*, 1991*a*). This approach differs fundamentally from other transgenic techniques in that the copy number remains unchanged, whereas the other approaches introduce extra copies of the gene under study into the genome of the mouse at random. Gene targeting via HR is therefore the most generally applicable method for testing whether human mutations are indeed pathogenic. Such models will clearly be invaluable for gaining a greater understanding of the pathogenesis of disease and for assessing targets for rational drug design. In diseases such as Alzheimer's disease and prion diseases where a minority of cases are genetic, a detailed study of gene-targeted animal models may enable the identification of biological markers of relevance to both the genetic and the sporadic forms of the disease.

Transgenic models of human diseases will also be useful in the development of gene therapy strategies to compensate for endogenous insufficiencies observed in disease. Some success has been reported in mice homozygous for the autosomal recessive shiverer mutation mapped to mouse chromosome 18 (Readhead *et al.*, 1987). These mice lack myelin basic protein (MBP) and have a characteristic phenotype of tremors, convulsions and early death. The wild type MBP gene has been introduced into the germline of shiverer mice by microinjection of fertilized eggs and the resulting transgenic mice no longer shiver or die prematurely.

Agriculture and medicine

The application of transgenic techniques has also been directed towards agriculture and is of potential economic importance. One goal is the production of disease-resistant animals, which may also have implications in human preventative medicine. A disease-resistant mouse model has been generated by microinjection of a fusion gene consisting of the metallothionein I gene promoter–regulatory region and the human β-1-interferon gene. Increased survival times were found in transgenic mice following pseudorabies virus challenge compared to their non-transgenic littermates. Also, sera from the transgenic mice protected human WISH cells from vesicular stomatitis virus infection (Chen, Yun & Wagner, 1988). Other studies have investigated methods of producing disease resistance in animals by creating transgenic mice resistant to the Moloney murine leukemia virus (M-MuLV). These mice express antisense RNA complementary to the retroviral packaging sequences by virtue of the integration into their germline of a construct containing the M-MuLV proviral packaging sequences in reverse orientation and under the control of the cytomegalovirus immediate-early region. The antisense RNA is thought to interfere with M-MuLV RNA and prevent encapsidation of genomic viral RNA, thus inhibiting viral replication (Han, Yun & Wagner, 1991).

Economically encouraged studies include the investigation of hair development in transgenic mice by the integration of a hair-specific murine ultra-high-sulphur keratin promoter fused to a chloramphenicol acetyltranferase reporter gene (McNab et al., 1990). Ultimately such studies may allow the manipulation of hair growth and density to improve wool production in sheep. The desire for greater meat production has led to considerable work being directed towards investigating growth hormone genes, their regulation, role in mammalian development and neuroendocrine effects. In many of these studies the inducible metallothionein I gene promoter is fused with a growth hormone gene. Mice transgenic for growth hormone can grow significantly larger than their non-transgenic littermates (Palmiter et al., 1982). Similar fusion genes have been successfully expressed in rabbits and pigs (Hammer et al., 1985). Limited success in terms of enhanced weight gain has been shown in these animals, although pigs expressing a bovine growth hormone fusion gene are reported to gain weight somewhat faster than controls.

An understanding of the promoter sequences required to induce expression during lactation in the mammal has led to the development of transgenesis in larger mammals (Clark et al., 1989). This is of particular importance for proteins that are otherwise derived from human blood and/or require complex post-translational processing that cannot be reproduced in cell culture systems. Production of proteins in mammals means that they will be correctly post-translationally modified, compared to expression of foreign genes in prokaryotic expression vectors. In addition, purification of the protein from milk is relatively easy. Similar transgenic experiments are now being carried out in goats and cattle, both of which produce more milk than a lactating sheep. Milk production is a prime target for the large-scale production of proteins. For example, sheep transgenic for the fusion gene, ovine β-lactoglobulin (sheep whey protein) gene promoter and human α-1-antitrypsin (hα1AT) produce active hα1AT that is indistinguishable from the human plasma-derived material (Wright *et al.*, 1991). A similar lactoglobulin promoter was combined with the human Factor XI (FXI) gene for FXI production in sheep milk (Clark *et al.*, 1989). Long-acting human tissue-type plasminogen activator (tPA) has been produced in the milk of transgenic goats by virtue of a murine whey acidic protein (WAP) promoter/human tPA fusion gene integrated into their germ-line (Ebert *et al.*, 1991).

Improvements in the composition of milk have been sought using transgenic techniques. Aims include the increase in the proportion of casein relative to the less useful whey proteins, the production of novel caseins such as those designed to improve the texture of cheeses and the heat stability of milk, and the possible production of bacteriocidal proteins in milk to combat mastitis.

Transgenic animals can also be used as models for toxicity testing. An example has been described in which transgenic mice expressing genes capable of repairing DNA have been generated to study the effect of DNA-damaging agents on tissue-specific carcinogenesis (Lim *et al.*, 1990). Similarly, a bacterio-phage lambda shuttle vector has been introduced into the mouse genome to generate a better predictor of long-term bioassay in whole animals and which included a mutagenicity assessment in germ cells (Kohler *et al.*, 1990). The vector contains a *lacZ* target gene, enabling scoring of mutations by colour assay when phage plaques incorporating the challenged transgenic mouse DNA are grown on indicator agar. This provides an *in vivo* assay of the mutagenic effects of chemicals.

New applications of transgenic technology are appearing in the literature with increasing rapidity. These have both economic importance to medicine and agriculture and biological importance to understanding the fundamental mechansims of normal development and disease processes.

References

Al-Shawi, R., Kinnaird, J., Burke, J. & Bishop, J. (1990). Expression of a foreign gene in a line of transgenic mice is modulated by a chromosomal position effect. *Molecular and Cellular Biology*, **10**, 1192–8.

Allen, N., Barton, S., Surani, A. & Reik, W. (1987). *Production of Transgenic Mice. A Practical Approach* (ed. M. Monk), pp. 217–34. IRL Press, Oxford.

Allen, N., Cran, D., Barton, S. *et al.* (1988). Transgenes as probes for active chromosomal domains in mouse development. *Nature*, **333**, 852–5.

Bradley, A., Evans, M., Kaufman, M. & Robertson, E. (1984). Formation of germ-line chimaeras from embryo-derived teratocarcinoma cell lines. *Nature*, **309**, 255–6.

Breitman, M., Clapoff, S., Rossant, J. *et al.* (1987). Genetic ablation: targeted expression of a toxin gene causes microphthalmia in transgenic mice. *Science*, **238**, 1563–5.

Brinster, R., Allen, J., Behringer, R. *et al.* (1988). Introns increase transcriptional efficiency in transgenic mice. *Proceedings of the National Academy of Sciences, USA*, **85**, 836–40.

Brinster, R., Chen, H., Trumbauer, M. *et al.* (1981). Somatic expression of Herpes thymidine kinase in mice following injection of a fusion gene into eggs. *Cell*, **27**, 223–31.

Brinster, R., Chen, H., Trumbauer, M. *et al.* (1985). Factors affecting the efficiency of introducing foreign DNA into mice by microinjecting eggs. *Proceedings of the National Academy of Sciences, USA*, **82**, 4438–42.

Capecchi, M. (1989). The new mouse genetics: altering the genome by gene targeting. *Trends in Genetics*, **5**, 70–6.

Chada, K., Magram, J., Raphael, K. *et al.* (1985). Specific expression of a foreign beta-globin gene in erythroid cells of transgenic mice. *Nature*, **314**, 377–80.

Chen, X.-Z., Yun, J. & Wagner, T. (1988). Enhanced viral resistance in transgenic mice expressing the human beta 1 interferon. *Journal of Virology*, **62**, 3883–7.

Choi, T., Huang, M., Gorman, C. & Jaenisch, R. (1991). A generic intron increases gene expression in transgenic mice. *Molecular and Cellular Biology*, **11**, 3070–4.

Clark, A., Ali, S., Archibald, A. *et al.* (1989). The molecular manipulation of milk composition. *Genome*, **31**, 950–5.

Costantini, P. & Lacy, E. (1981). Introduction of a rabbit beta-globin gene into the mouse germline. *Nature*, **294**, 92–4.

Doetschman, T., Gregg, R., Maeda, N. *et al.* (1987). Targetted correction of a mutant HPRT gene in mouse embryonic stem cells. *Nature*, **330**, 576–8.

Ebert, K., Selgrath, J., DiTullio, P. *et al.* (1991). Transgenic production of a variant of human tissue-type plasminogen activator in goat milk: generation of transgenic goats and analysis of expression. *Biotechnology*, **9**, 835–7.

Evans, M. & Kaufman, M. (1981). Establishment in culture of pluripotential cells from mouse embryos. *Nature*, **292**, 154–6.

Forss-Petter, S., Danielson, P., Catsicas, S. *et al.* (1990). Transgenic mice expressing beta-galactosidase in mature neurons under neuron-specific enolase promoter control. *Neuron*, **5**, 187–97.

Gordon, J., Chesa, P., Nishimura, H. *et al.* (1987). Regulation of Thy-1 gene expression in transgenic mice. *Cell*, **50**, 445–52.

Goring, D., Rossant, J., Clapoff, S. *et al.* (1987). In situ detection of β-galactosidase in lenses of transgenic mice with a γ-crystallin/lacZ gene. *Science*, **244**, 463–5.

Gossler, A., Joyner, A., Rossant, J. & Skarnes, D. (1989). Mouse embryonic stem cells and reporter constructs to detect developmentally regulated genes. *Science*, **244**, 463–5.

Hammer, R., Krumlauf, R., Camper, S. *et al.* (1987). Diversity of α-fetoprotein gene expression in mice is generated by a combination of separate enhancer elements. *Science*, **235**, 53–8.

Hammer, R., Pursel, V., Rexroad, C. *et al.* (1985). Production of transgenic rabbits, sheep and pigs by microinjection. *Nature*, **315**, 680–3.

Han, L., Yun, J. & Wagner, T. (1991). Inhibition of Moloney murine leukemia virus-induced leukemia in transgenic mice expressing antisense RNA complementary to the retroviral packaging sequences. *Proceedings of the National Academy of Sciences, USA*, **88**, 4313–17.

Hasty, P., Ramirez-Solis, R., Krumlauf, R. & Bradley, A. (1991*a*). Introduction of a subtle mutation into the Hox-2.6 locus in embryonic stem cells. *Nature*, **350**, 243–6.

Hasty, P., Rivera-Perez, J. & Bradley, A. (1991*b*). The length of homology required for gene targeting in embryonic stem cells. *Molecular Cellular Biology*, **11**, 5586–91.

Hasty, P., Rivera-Perez, J., Chang, C. & Bradley, A. (1991*c*). Target frequency and integration pattern for insertion and replacement vectors in embryonic stem cells. *Molecular Cellular Biology*, **11**, 4509–17.

Hogan, B., Constantini, F. & Lacy, E. (1986). *Manipulating the mouse embryo: a laboratory manual*. Cold Spring Harbor Laboratory Press, New York.

Hsiao, K., Scott, M., Foster, D. *et al.* (1990). Spontaneous neurodegeneration in transgenic mice with mutant prion protein. *Science*, **250**, 1587–90.

Jaenisch, R. (1976). Germ line integration and Mendelian transmission of the exogenous Moloney leukemia virus. *Proceedings of the National Academy of Sciences, USA*, **73**, 1260–9.

Jaenisch, R., Jahner, D., Nobis, P. *et al.* (1981). Chromosomal position and activation of retroviral genomes inserted into the germline of mice. *Cell*, **24**, 519–29.

Jahner, D., Haase, K., Mulligan, R. & Jaenisch, R. (1985). Insertion of the bacterial gpt gene into the germline of mice by retroviral infection. *Proceedings of the National Academy of Sciences, USA*, **82**, 6927–31.

Jasin, M. & Berg, P. (1988). Homologous integration in mammalian cells without target gene selection. *Genes & Development*, **2**, 1353–63.

Jeannotte, L., Ruiz, J. & Robertson, E. (1991). Low level of Hox1.3 gene expression does not preclude the use of promoterless vectors to generate a targeted gene disruption. *Molecular Cellular Biology*, **11**, 5578–85.

Joyner, A., Skarnes, W. & Rossant, J. (1989). Production of a mutation in the mouse En-2 gene by homologous recombination in embryonic stem cells. *Nature*, **338**, 153–6.

Kawabata, S., Higgins, G. A. & Gordon, J. W. (1991). Amyloid plaques, neurofibrillary tangles, and neuronal loss in brains of transgenic mice overexpressing a C-terminal fragment of human amyloid precursor protein in neurons of the central nervous system. *Nature*, **354**, 476–8.

Kim, H. & Smithies, O. (1988). Recombinant fragment assay for gene targeting based on the polymerase chain reaction. *Nucleic Acids Research*, **16**, 8887–903.

Kohler, S., Provost, G., Kretz, P. *et al.* (1990). The use of transgenic mice for short-term, in vivo mutagenicity testing. *Genetic Analysis Techniques and Applications*, **7**, 212–18.

Koller, B., Hagemann, L., Doetschman, T. *et al.* (1989). Germ-line transmission of a planned alteration made in a hypoxanthine phosphoribosyltransferase gene by homologous recombination in embryonic stem cells. *Proceedings of the National Academy of Sciences, USA*, **86**, 8927–31.

Kothary, R., Clapoff, S., Brown, A. *et al.* (1988). A transgene containing *lacZ* inserted into the *dystonia* locus is expressed in neural tube. *Nature*, **335**, 435–7.

Lim, I., Dumenco, L., Yun, J. *et al.* (1990). High level, regulated expression of the chimeric P-enolpyruvate carboxykinase (GTP)-bacterial O^6-alkylguanine-DNA alkyltransferase (*ada*) gene in transgenic mice. *Cancer Research*, **50**, 1701–8.

Mansour, S., Thomas, K. & Capecchi, M. (1988). Disruption of the proto-oncogene int-2 in mouse embryonic stem cells: a general strategy for targeting mutations to non-selectable genes. *Nature*, **336**, 348–52.

Martin, G. (1981). Isolation of a pluripotent cell line from early mouse embryos cultured in medium conditioned by teratocarcinoma stem cells. *Proceedings of the National Academy of Sciences, USA*, **78**, 7634–8.

McMahon, A. & Bradley, A. (1990). The Wnt 1 proto oncogene is required for development of a large region of the mouse brain. *Cell*, **62**, 1073–85.

McNab, A., Andrus, P., Wagner, T. *et al.* (1990). Hair-specific expression of chloramphenicol acetyltransferase in transgenic mice under the control of a ultra-high-sulfur keratin promoter. *Proceedings of the National Academy of Sciences, USA*, **87**, 6848–52.

Meyer, K., Sharpe, M., Surani, M. & Neuberger, M. (1990). The importance of the 3′-enhancer region in immunoglobulin k gene expression. *Nucleic Acids Research*, **18**, 5609–15.

Palmiter, R., Behringer, R., Quaife, C. *et al.* (1987). Cell lineage ablation in transgenic mice by cell-specific expression of a toxin gene. *Cell*, **50**, 435–43.

Palmiter, R. & Brinster, R. (1986). Transgenic mice. *Annual Reviews of Genetics*, **20**, 465–99.

Palmiter, R., Brinster, R., Hammer, R. *et al.* (1982). Dramatic growth of mice that develop from eggs microinjected with metallothionein-growth hormone fusion genes. *Nature*, **300**, 611–15.

Palmiter, R., Sandgren, E., Avarbock, M. *et al.* (1991). Heterologous introns can enhance gene expression of transgenes in mice. *Proceedings of the National Academy of Sciences, USA*, **88**, 478–82.

Prusiner, S. B., Scott, M., Foster, D. *et al.* (1990). Transgenetic studies implicate interactions between homologous PrP isoforms in scrapie prion replication. *Cell*, **63**, 673–6.

Quon, D., Wang, Y., Catalano, R. *et al.* (1991). Formation of β-amyloid protein deposits in brains of transgenic mice. *Nature*, **352**, 239–41.

Raich, N., Enver, T., Nakamoto, B. *et al.* (1990). Autonomous developmental control of human embryonic globin gene switching in transgenic mice. *Science*, **250**, 1147–9.

Readhead, C., Popko, B., Takahashi, N. *et al.* (1987). Expression of a myelin basic protein gene in transgenic *Shiverer* mice: correction of the dysmyelinating phenotype. *Cell*, **48**, 703–12.

Reeves, R., Pavan, W. & Hieter, P. (1990). Modification and manipulation of mammalian DNA cloned as YACs. *Genetic Analysis Techniques and Applications*, **7**, 107–13.

Robertson, E., Bradley, A., Kuehn, M. & Evans, M. (1986). Germline transmission of genes introduced into cultured pluripotential cells by retroviral vector. *Nature*, **323**, 445–8.

Schwartzberg, P., Goff, S. & Robertson, E. (1989). Germ-line transmission of a c-abl mutation produced by targeted gene disruption in ES cells. *Science*, **246**, 799–804.

Scott, M., Foster, M., Mirenda, C. *et al.* (1989). Transgenic mice expressing hamster prion protein produce species-specific scrapie infectivity and amyloid plaques. *Cell*, **59**, 847–57.

Shih, D., Wall, R. & Shapiro, S. (1990). Developmentally regulated and erythroid-specific expression of the human embryonic beta-globin gene in transgenic mice. *Nucleic Acids Research*, **18**, 5465–72.

Stamatoyannopoulos, G. (1991). Human hemoglobin switching. *Science*, **252**, 383.

Swain, J., Stewart, T. & Leder, P. (1987). Parental legacy determines methylation and expression of an autosomal transgene: a molecular mechanism for parental imprinting. *Cell*, **70**, 719–27.

Swift, J. & Hammer, R. (1984). Tissue-specific expression of the rat pancreatic elastase 1 gene in transgenic mice. *Cell*, **38**, 639–46.

Thomas, K. & Capecchi, M. (1987). Site-directed mutagenesis by gene targeting in mouse embryo-derived stem cells. *Cell*, **51**, 503–12.

Townes, T., Lingrel, J., Chen, H. *et al.* (1985). Erythroid specific expression of human beta-globin genes in transgenic mice. *EMBO Journal*, **4**, 1715–23.

Trudel, M. & Costantini, F. (1987). A 3' enhancer contributes to the stage-specific expression of the human beta-globin gene. *Genes and Development*, **1**, 954–61.

van der Putten, H., Botteri, F., Miller, A. *et al.* (1985). Efficient insertion of genes into the mouse germ-line via retroviral vectors. *Proceedings of the National Academy of Sciences, USA*, **82**, 6148–52.

Wirak, D. O., Bayney, R., Kundel, C. A. *et al.* (1991*a*). Regulatory region of human amyloid precursor protein (APP) gene promotes neuron-specific gene expression in the CNS of transgenic mice. *EMBO Journal*, **10**, 289–96.

Wirak, D. O., Bayney, R., Ramaghadran, T. V. *et al.* (1991*b*). Deposits of amyloid-protein in the central nervous system of transgenic mice. *Science*, **253**, 323–5.

Woychik, R., Stewart, J., Davis, L. *et al.* (1985). An inherited limb deformity created by insertional mutagenesis in a transgenic mouse. *Nature*, **318**, 36–40.

Wright, G., Carver, A., Cottom, D. *et al.* (1991). High level expression of active human alpha-1-antitrypsin in the milk of transgenic sheep. *Biotechnology*, **9**, 830–4.

Zimmer, A. & Gruss, P. (1989). Production of chimaeric mice containing ES cells carrying a homeo-box Hox 1.1 allele mutated by homologous recombination. *Nature*, **338**, 150–2.

Note added in proof

A new transgenic technique has recently been developed using the Cre-loxP site-specific recombination system derived from bacteriophage. This system allows the introduction of mutations into the mouse genome in a cell-type specific manner. Mutations that would normally produce a lethal phenotype can now be studied as the mutant animals produced in this manner are viable.

Gu, H., Marth, J. D., Orban, P. C., Mossmann, H. & Rajewsky, K. (1994). Deletion of a DNA polymerase β gene segment in T-cells using cell type-specific gene targeting. *Science*, **265**, 103–6.

11

Neuropathology by numbers: application of image analysis techniques to quantitative neuropathology

M. CLAIRE ROYSTON

Traditional examination or evaluation of neuropathological material involves visual inspection with the expectation of identifying and/or classifying the items of interest within the specimen. Recent refinements of classical histological staining techniques and the emergence of immunocytochemistry as a powerful investigative tool in neuropathology have considerably widened not only the scope of the histological material studied but also the types of information that are sought from the material. Manual visual methods involve the complex and skilled procedure of interpreting a microscopic image together with a series of subjective decisions in order to determine if a particular feature, for example tumour cells, is present, thereby enabling a diagnosis to be made. However, in addition to the function of making a diagnosis, quantitative neuropathology is increasingly being adopted to study the molecular mechanisms that culminate in the end-state gross pathological features of a disorder. Here the issue extends beyond identifying the presence of a pathological lesion to much more complex questions concerning quantitative descriptions of the *number* or *spatial arrangement* of a particular feature. For example, one might ask what is the ratio of classic to diffuse β/A4 protein positive plaques in cases of Alzheimer's disease with differing aetiological antecedents, or what is the laminar arrangement of the β/A4 deposition within key cortical areas.

The subjective elements inherent in manual techniques have been shown to introduce a divergence in diagnostic categorization (e.g. Childhood Brain Tumour Consortium, 1989). However, when more complex quantitative questions are asked, involving many more subjective decisions, there is a concomitant increase in the degree of inconsistency. For example, a difference of up to 25% between raters was noted when a series of experienced neuropathologists attended to the plaque classification question (Mirra *et al.*, 1990).

In order to circumvent these difficulties and to undertake the examination of the vast numbers of sections that are generated in many experiments computerized image analysis is increasingly being employed in quantitative neuropathological studies. One further advantage of image analysis that is only just beginning to be recognized is its potential to examine and quantify fundamental aspects of a histological image that are not readily accessible to the human investigator, for example the characteristic components of a colour image, such as saturation relating to stain purity, hue representing the principal wavelength and intensity (Julis & Mikes, 1992) or the fractal dimensions of cellular profiles (Smith *et al.*, 1989).

Image analysis at its simplest level may be defined as *the numerical description of images*; in more detail, it encompasses a range of mathematical techniques that allow us to ascribe a number to a particular facet of an image in terms of number of elements, for example size, shape and spatial arrangement and thereby compare these features between different individuals or in different experimental conditions.

As image analysis systems become both more sophisticated and relatively less costly, image analysis methods are being utilized more and more in neuropathological studies of the brain. Image analysis techniques are increasingly being used to analyse data from a wide range of neuroscience studies *in vivo* – magnetic resonance imaging (e.g. Schaefer *et al.*, 1990), CT scanning (e.g. Casanova *et al.*, 1989) and positron emission tomography (e.g. Friston *et al.*, 1990). *In vitro* techniques utilizing image analysis include autoradiography (e.g. Royston *et al.*, 1991), cell culture and *in situ* hybridization (de Belleroche *et al.*, 1990). This chapter, however, will focus on image analysis techniques as applied to examining histological preparations of the brain using immunocytochemical staining techniques (see Chapter 5). The topic will be considered under three sub-headings: first, the basic components of an image analysis system are reviewed, second, the underlying principles in designing an experimental protocol are considered, finally, a series of illustrations of the application of image analysis to examine specific neuropathological questions are presented.

Basic components of an image analysis system

The basic functions of an image analysis system are simple, although the hardware and software necessary to realize these functions are sophisticated. In principle, an image analysis system, whether PC or mainframe based, has four main elements

> **video camera** inputs the image to the system
> **framestore** converts camera output to digital format
> **monitor** views the digitized image
> **software** allows measurements to be made

These features are combined with a keyboard or mouse to interact with the image and computing facility, computer memory to store (archive) the images and some form of output device (for example, printer) to deliver results. In neuropathology, there is the additional requirement of a microscope to deliver the microscopic image to the video camera. Figure 11.1 shows an example of a commercially available system.

Essentially two different types of camera have been incorporated into image analysis systems – tube cameras and solid-state CCD (charge coupled) cameras. In recent years there has been an 'explosion' in camera technology and high-quality cameras that deliver a stable and reliable image into the system are readily available at reasonable cost. The rapid developments have in the main been in the field of CCD cameras, which have the advantage, compared to tube cameras, of higher resolution and significantly less distortion of the image. However, in atypical lighting conditions, for example very low light level or infra-red, then a tube camera may be preferable.

The range of analytical functions possible using the software contained within a given image analyser system varies considerably with machines from a range of different manufacturers. Unfortunately, when image analysis is applied to neuropathology, machines are not supplied with a 'counting neurones' function. What is available are basic algorithms that can be built up in a 'tool-box' manner, which allow the development of a routine tailored to a particular application. Examples of such routines are presented in detail in the last section of this chapter.

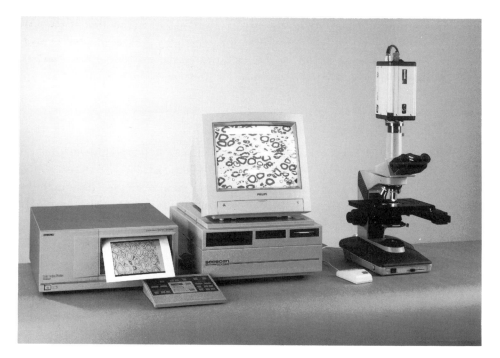

Figure 11.1. Example of a commercially available image analysis system. Photograph courtesy of Seescan PLC, Cambridge, UK.

Designing an experimental protocol

This can be broken down into four basic steps, each of which has a number of commonly met pitfalls, which will be discussed in this section. It is fundamental to recognize that image analysis is a tool and that in order to use the tool sensibly the first prerequisite is to have a pertinent question or application to investigate. The basic steps are:

sample preparation
image acquisition and processing
measurements
treatment of results

Sample preparation

This aspect of image analysis often receives scant attention, however, it remains one of the most important determinants of a valid and meaningful result. Irrespective of the complexity of the subsequent image processing and analysis, if poor-quality samples are used then the experimental outcome cannot be relied upon. Some basic points are as follows:

Material

Preliminary experiments should be undertaken to investigate the effects of potential confounding variables on the extent of the material's reaction with the stain used, for example the effect of age, agonal state, or post-mortem delay. Hence material matched to account for these features is desirable.

Section preparation

It is important that sections of a uniform thickness are used throughout an experiment. In, for example, a 15 μm section immunostained with an antibody to β/A4 protein, what is actually visualized is a two-dimensional projection of the immuno-positive elements in a three-dimensional block of material; clearly this cannot be meaningfully compared with a section that is 30 μm wide, where an increased area of projected stained elements may not necessarily represent an increase in the absolute 'amount' of β/A4 protein deposited in the cortex.

Staining of sections

Immunocytochemical staining rests on a simple principle of using antibodies directed against specific antigens of interest, which are visualized by chromogens that produce a coloured reaction product. The amount of reaction product visualized depends on the amount of antigen present (that is, the item of interest) and is also critically dependent on the concentrations of the reagents used in the experiment. Thus, in order to make a valid interpretation of results it is important that all staining should follow an established protocol detailing the precise concentration of reagents, in carefully controlled conditions. It is therefore desirable that all sections within a given experiment are stained in the same staining 'run'.

Immunocytochemistry has many advantages in terms of the specificity of staining, using carefully raised monoclonal antibodies, and the level of detailed resolution of individually labelled cells and fibres that can be studied. However, it is not an absolute technique so that serial sections may not stain to the same intensity in two separate experiments. However, a linear relationship has been demonstrated between the concentration of an antigen and the optical density produced by immunocytochemical labelling of an antibody raised against the antigen (Nabours, Songu-Mize & Mize, 1988). Radioimmunoassay techniques have also been used to validate quantitative immunocytochemistry (e.g. Benno *et al.*, 1982).

Image acquisition and processing

Acquisition and processing covers all the stages involved in presenting an image to the digitizer within the image analyser and the manipulation of image to allow the desired measurements to be made. The first stage in this process is at the level of the microscope. Here the nature of the image presented to the camera is very dependent on the optical characteristics and settings of the microscope and also on the level and consistency of the light source illuminating the microscopic section. Care must be taken to ensure that these features are optimized and held constant throughout an experiment.

In digitizing the image, a number of phenomena occur. It is important to consider these in relation to the type of information that is subsequently sought from the image. The light-sensitive elements within the CCD camera – termed pixels – enable the camera to transmit an image (as an analogue signal) to the framestore, which converts the signal to a digital format using an analogue digital converter, and it can then be stored as a number array. The process of digitization may thus be likened to recreating the *continuous* image as a *discontinuous* image akin to a mosaic. This introduces the important concept of spatial resolution; clearly the size and shape of the 'bricks' – pixels – that the mosaic is composed of will influence the clarity and detail that is available in the digitized image. Items that are smaller than an individual pixel will be lost as information in the digitized image. Another, very pertinent, issue in neuropathological studies, is that two-dimensional profile of many items of interest in neuropathology, for example a cell is roughly circular, are 'reproduced' in the digitized image using rectangular pixel elements. If the question asked is 'what is the area of the cells?' then the error introduced using the digitized representation of the circular profile will be proportionately greater the smaller the overall profile – that is, the fewer pixels the profile covers. This problem can be circumvented by decreasing the size of each pixel (1024 by 1024), but this often introduces a lot of 'noise' into the image. The preferred manoeuvre would be to increase the magnification of the image so that the number of pixels covered by the boundary of the profile, which can potentially contribute to the error, are relatively reduced in comparison to the total area of the overall profile.

In addition to spatial information, a digitized image contains data representing the brightness of the image. Information is encoded in relation to a discrete grey-scale. Again, the number of divisions between black and white that the machine can recognize will have a direct effect on the detail of the returned image. It is noteworthy that the human eye can theoretically recognize approximately 64 separate grey levels compared to the standard grey-scale used with CCD cameras, which can recognize 256 separate grey levels. As a practical note, it is important to quote both features of a system, for example spatial resolution of 512 by 512 pixels with a 256 grey-shade scale, when reporting the results of an experiment.

In neuropathological studies we are frequently examining cells or features of a section that are stained dark against a pale background and it is this feature that allows the image to be segmented or thresholded (sub-divided) into item and non-item or background. Considerable advantage can be gained by refining immunostaining protocols to produce high contrast images allowing easier segmentation (e.g. Gentleman *et al.*, 1989). In an ideal situation there would be a precise grey level (in terms of a lower and upper value) that isolated the item of interest from background grey levels, reflecting maximal contrast between item and background. These theoretical points could then be identified and the image analyser 'told' to ignore those parts of the image that lay outside these boundaries. However, in practice these points are difficult to identify and two approaches have been adopted to select appropriate threshold levels. So-called automated threshold settings are usually based on probability predictions, based on grey-level frequency histograms (e.g. Bruce *et al.*, 1992). The alternative approach is to use interactive techniques, which necessitate the user setting the grey levels based on the visual inspection of the image. Reliable interactive thresholding can be achieved if detailed operationalized criteria are established prior to the experiment (e.g. Edwards *et al.*, 1992). Once again, it should be appreciated that the image analysis process will have a direct effect upon the accuracy and reliability of even a simple question such as 'what is the area covered by a dark-staining element in a given image?'. If wide grey levels are selected, there is the possibility that more pixels will be included within the thresholded items and give a higher area measurement compared to the same image thresholded using narrower grey-level settings. It is therefore of paramount importance that considerable care is spent in determining, for each experimental procedure, precisely how the image will be thresholded and that what is selected as item corresponds to what can be seen in the microscopic image. Details of the reliability (both intra and inter rater) should be presented when a novel image-analysis protocol is proposed.

The last stage in image processing involves 'optimizing' the digitized image to enable information to be extracted. This includes a number of standard algorithms to remove 'noise' from an image, for example any dark-stained elements which are constituted only by a single pixel, together with routines that will enhance contrast within an image by using filters or smoothing operations. Sophisticated algorithms are currently being developed and validated to separate overlapping items within an image or to allow an X-profile to be correctly identified as two separate crossed fibres rather than a single X-shaped fibre. A further frequently adopted measure to enhance the contrast within an image is to subtract an image of only background staining (for example, white matter staining when examining immunostained neuronal cell bodies) from the raw image to return a processed image reflecting staining intensity of the neuronal elements, separated from staining intensity from non-specific aggregation of reaction product.

Measurements

Having obtained an image that can be studied, the question of what measurements are to be made arises. These will be dictated by the hypothesis the experiment is designed to address and, as mentioned earlier, if there is no question there can be no answer. At a basic level two types of measurements, object measurements and field measurements, can be made.

Object measurements

Number
This may be a total count of items per slide, but more usually represents counts in a series of microscopic fields. In the latter case numerical density values are more robust, for example neurones per mm^2 cortex.

Simple geometric properties
Here features such as the length, circumference or cross-sectional area of items may be compared.

Derived geometric properties
More complex features such as shape factor, which is the ratio of area of an item to $perimeter^2$, may be used to differentiate items. Using this definition, 1 represents a perfect circle and at the opposite extreme 0 represents a straight line.

Spatial arrangement

Items within a field have definable relationship to each other and to other features that may be of interest, for example orientation of cells or relative position and distribution of neurones within the cortex.

Field measurements

Proportion of field stained

Within a thresholded image, a calibrated measuring frame may be used to determine the simple ratio (area stained element/area sampled), or expressed as a 'load' measurement defined as % of region occupied by stained elements.

Optical density

The amount of light transmitted through a specimen can be expressed as transmittance, which is defined as ratio of transmitted to incident light. The other term frequently used is optical density, which is the amount of incident light that has been attenuated by the specimen

$$\text{density} = \log_{10} 1/\text{transmittance}$$

The majority of image-analysis machines have algorithms to compute these features. In order to 'create' an image analysis protocol, those features of interest are selected. To make the selection one must examine the question that is being addressed by the experiment.

Application of image analysis to quantitative neuropathology

One of the first obstacles to be overcome is the issue of sampling. Even if a very sophisticated image analysis routine is developed to quantify, for example, numerical density of neuronal cell bodies in a specific area of cortex, the outcome of the experiment may be fundamentally distorted by a poor or biased sampling scheme. Sampling schemes have several important features:

random versus systematic
pattern design of scheme
number of samples per subject

Systematic sampling schemes have a number of theoretical advantages in relation to reduced level of bias and increased efficiency (see Gunderson & Jensen, 1987). However, in practice it is often difficult to secure material that satisfies all the requirements for these approaches. In quantifying the number of neurones within a sub-field of the hippocampus one may not have available more than a limited number of sections from which to work. Therefore, one has to adopt a random sampling scheme using the material that is available. Here one should be guided by what is already known about the distribution of the item to be quantified and what is known about the anatomical relationships and boundaries in the material as a whole. In designing a sampling scheme to examine the distribution of β/A4 positive plaques in the cortex, two factors were taken into consideration:

1. That the cortex is sub-divided into laminae and that these are very important functional and morphological delineations.
2. That the cytoarchitecture of the cortex is more complicated at the points of inflection at the bottom of sulci than at the relatively uniform extent of the gyri.

Hence a 'cortical strip' sampling scheme was adopted in which contiguous sampling frames were used to traverse the cortical thickness from pial surface to white matter interface; three strips were used at the crest of each gyrus.

Finally, there is the question of how many samples constitute a 'fair' sample; there is no simple answer to this question. Common sense indicates that if the overall surface area of subject matter is 1 cm^2 then sampling five microscopic fields at a magnification of $\times 40$ will not yield a very reliable result. The 'correct' number of samples will depend on the overall frequency of the item studied and its pattern of distribution.

There follows a series of examples, illustrating how we have used the image analysis techniques discussed in this chapter to examine specific questions in neuropathological research.

Example 1: Classification and quantification of plaque types in Alzheimer's disease using computerized image analysis (Edwards *et al.*, 1992)

In this study, the aim was to develop a reliable technique to objectively quantify the number of classic versus diffuse β/A4 plaques. Data from previous studies has been very inconsistent and difficult to interpret, owing to the variety of subjective classification criteria used within the studies. The β/A4 plaques were visualized by immunostaining and a series of mathematical criteria developed to differentiate between the two plaque types. These were based on the degree of roundness (classic plaques were more circular), texture (classic plaques have a more uniform density of staining) and the presence of a non-staining internal area (more likely in classic plaques). A discriminant function analysis was used to determine how well the combination of these three features were able to differentiate the two plaque types. In a 'test' experiment a misclassification rate of 9% was recorded; taken in context of a published error rate of 25% using visual inspection this compares very favourably (Mirra *et al.*, 1990). Using this methodology, we have been able to show that the number of classic versus diffuse plaques differs between sulci and gyri (McKenzie *et al.*, 1992) and also correlates significantly with the severity of dementia in patients with Down's syndrome (Royston *et al.*, 1994).

Example 2: Quantifying the pattern of β/A4 amyloid protein distribution in Alzheimer's disease by image analysis (Bruce *et al.*, 1992)

In this study the aim was to develop a technique that could be used to quantify the pattern of β/A4 protein distribution across the cortex and to compare this in different cortical areas. Forty equispaced measurements (area covered by thresholded elements/area measuring frame) were made along an axis orientated perpendicular to the pial surface and spanning the entire extent of the pial surface to white matter interface. A series of curves could therefore be constructed relating β/A4 distribution to distance across the cortex. The data from each of these curves was used to calculate a mathematical descriptor of the shape of the curve using sequential harmonic analysis (Royston *et al.*, 1991). We have now demonstrated a fundamental difference in the amyloid distribution pattern between the sulci and gyri, which may reflect the difference in the underlying cytoarchitecture of the cortex (Clinton *et al.*, 1993*b*).

Example 3: Relative synaptic index – assessment of synaptic density using synaptophysin immunocytochemistry and computerized image analysis (Clinton *et al.*, 1993*a*)

The methodology in this study was developed in order to permit the rapid and accurate assessment of synaptic density in human post-mortem material, to facilitate the study of synaptic pattern in a range of neuropsychiatric diseases. The synapse was visualized using synaptophysin – a pre-synaptic vesicle marker – thus giving an *relative* index of the synapse. Synaptophysin staining was quantified by optical density measurements and the paper presents details of both inter- and intra-rater reliability studies. Using this methodology, we have been able to demonstrate a significant difference in the relative synaptic index between different functional sub-divisions of the brain.

References

Benno, R. H., Tucker, L. W., Joh, T. H. & Reis, D. J. (1982). Quantitative immuno-cytochemistry of tyrosine hydroxylase in rat brain. I. Development of a computerised assisted method using the peroxidase-antiperoxidase technique. *Brain Research*, **246**, 225–36.

Barrett, A. J., Davies, M. E. & Grubb, A. (1984). The place of human γ-trace (cystatin C) amongst the cysteine proteinase inhibitors. *Biochemical and Biophysical Research Communications*, **120**, 631–6.

Bruce, C. V., Clinton, J., Gentleman, S. M. *et al.* (1992). Quantifying the pattern of amyloid distribution by image analysis. *Neuropathology and Applied Neurobiology*, **18**, 125–36.

Butler, E. A. & Flynn, F. V. (1961). The occurrence of post-gamma protein in urine: a new protein abnormality. *Journal of Clinical Pathology*, **14**, 172–8.

Casanova, M. F., Daniel, D. G., Goldberg, T. E. *et al.* (1989). Shape analysis of the middle cranial fossa of schizophrenic patients. A computerised tomographic study. *Schizophrenia Research*, **2**, 333–8.

Childhood Brain Tumour Consortium. (1989). Intra observer reproducibility in assigning brain tumours to classes in the World Health Organisation diagnostic scheme. *Journal of Neuro-Oncology*, **7**, 211–24.

Clinton, J., Forsythe, C., Royston, M. C. & Roberts, G. W. (1993). Synaptic degeneration is the primary neuropathological feature in prion disease: a preliminary study. *Neuroreport*, **4**, 65–8.

Clinton, J., Roberts, G. W., Gentleman, S. M. & Royston, M. C. (1993*b*). Differential pattern of β amyloid protein deposition within cortical sulci and gyri in Alzheimer's disease. *Neuropathology and Applied Neurobiology*, **19**, 277–81.

de Belleroche, J., Bandopadhyay, R., King, A. *et al.* (1990). Regional distribution of cholecystokinin messenger RNA in rat brain during development: quantitation and correlation with cholecystokinin immunoreactivity. *Neuropeptides*, **15**, 201–12.

Edwards, R. J., Clinton, J., Gentleman, S. M. *et al.* (1992). Classification and quantification of plaque types in Alzheimer's disease using computerised image analysis. *Neurodegeneration*, **1**, 65–71.

Friston, K. J., Frith, C. D., Liddle, P. F. *et al.* (1990). The relationship between global and local changes in PET scans. *Journal Cerebral Blood Flow and Metabolism*, **10**, 458–66.

Gentleman, S. M., Allsop, D., Bruton, C. J. *et al.* (1989). A demonstration of the advantages of immunostaining in the quantification of amyloid plaque deposits. *Histochemistry*, **92**, 355–8.

Gunderson, H. J. G. & Jensen, E. B. (1987). The efficiency of systematic sampling and its prediction. *Journal of Microscopy*, **147**, 229–63.

Julis, I. & Mikes, J. (1992). True colour image analysis and histopathology. *Microscopy and Analysis*, **30**, 9–11.

McKenzie, J. E., Gentleman, S. M., Royston, M. C. *et al.* (1992). Quantification of plaque types in sulci and gyri of the medical frontal lobe in patients with Alzheimer's disease. *Neuroscience Letters*, **143**, 23–6.

Mirra, S. S., Hughes, J. P., Van Belle, G. *et al.* (1990). The neuropathological evaluation of Alzheimer's disease: a multi-centre quality assurance study conducted by the Consortium to establish a Registry for Alzheimer's disease. *XIth International Congress of Neuropathology Abstracts*, p. 183.

Nabours, B. L., Songu-Mize, E. & Mize, R. R. (1988). Quantitative immuno-cytochemistry using an image analyzer. II. Concentration standards for transmitter immunocytochemistry. *Journal of Neuroscience Methods*, **26**, 25–34.

Royston, M. C., Kodical, N. F., Mann, D. M. A. & Groom, K. (1994). Quantitative analysis of β-amyloid deposition in Down's Syndrome using computerised image analysis. *Neurodegeneration*, **3**, 43–51.

Royston, M. C., Slater, P., Simpson, M. D. C. & Deakin, J. F. W. (1991). Analysis of laminar distribution of kappa opiate receptors in human cortex: comparison between schizophrenia and normal. *Journal of Neuroscience Methods*, **36**, 145–53.

Schaefer, G. B., Thompson, J. N., Bodensteiner, J. B. *et al.* (1990). Quantitative morphometric analysis of brain growth using magnetic resonance imaging. *Journal of Child Neurology*, **5**, 127–30.

Smith, T. G., Marks, W. B., Lange, G. D. *et al.* (1989). A fractal analysis of cell images. *Journal of Neuroscience Methods*, **27**, 173–80.

Index